ALCOHOL AND
HUMAN MEMORY

ALCOHOL AND HUMAN MEMORY

Edited by
ISABEL M. BIRNBAUM
UNIVERSITY OF CALIFORNIA, IRVINE

ELIZABETH S. PARKER
NATIONAL INSTITUTE ON ALCOHOL ABUSE
AND ALCOHOLISM

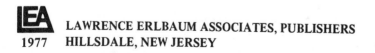

LAWRENCE ERLBAUM ASSOCIATES, PUBLISHERS
1977   HILLSDALE, NEW JERSEY

DISTRIBUTED BY THE HALSTED PRESS DIVISION OF

JOHN WILEY & SONS

New York   Toronto   London   Sydney

Lawrence Erlbaum Associates, Inc., Publishers
62 Maria Drive
Hillsdale, New Jersey 07642

Distributed solely by Halsted Press Division
John Wiley & Sons, Inc., New York

Library of Congress Cataloging in Publication Data

Main entry under title:

Alcohol and human memory.

 Papers presented at a conference sponsored by the
National Institute on Alcohol Abuse and Alcoholism,
Sept. 9-10, 1976, in Laguna Beach, Calif.
 Includes bibliographical references.
 1. Alcoholism–Congresses. 2. Alcohol–Physiological
effect–Congresses. 3. Memory–Congresses.
I. Birnbaum, Isabel M. II. Parker, Elizabeth S.
III. National Institute on Alcohol and Alcoholism.
RC565.A39 616.8'61'07 77-15653
ISBN 0-470-99339-1

Printed in the United States of America

Contents

Foreword

Alcohol abuse constitutes the third greatest health problem in the United States today. An estimated 9 million people are alcoholic or problem drinkers, and this number appears to be on the rise. There is an urgent need to improve current efforts toward preventing and treating alcohol-related problems. To maximize the effectiveness of these efforts, a base of reliable, objective, and scientific facts needs to be established.

The National Institute on Alcohol Abuse and Alcoholism places a high priority on research. Through the development of excellent research it is possible to answer some of the crucial and fundamental questions about alcohol. Even though the subject of alcohol abuse is exceedingly complex, it is imperative that probing questions continue to be asked. Thus, the NIAAA is encouraging scientists at the forefront of their respective areas of scientific inquiry to apply their expertise to advance our knowledge about the actions of alcohol.

This volume illustrates the significant benefits that evolve through interdisciplinary research. Some of the significant strides being made in understanding the ways alcohol alters cognitive processes are highlighted in the following chapters, as are many of the exciting new directions in which research in this area will proceed.

Memory is one of the most important human attributes. That alcohol, a drug, when given acutely or chronically can impair memory is a fact worthy of our most serious attention. In-depth knowledge of alcohol's effects on memory could lead to a better understanding of the vicious cycles of drinking and other aberrant behaviors that alcoholics experience. This is a challenging area for investigation, and we must proceed in the spirit of excellence.

ERNEST P. NOBLE*
*Director, National Institute on
Alcohol Abuse and Alcoholism*

*This foreword was prepared by Ernest P. Noble in his private capacity. No official support or endorsement by the ADAMHA or NIAAA is intended or should be inferred.

Preface

The papers in this volume were presented at a conference on Alcohol and Memory sponsored by the National Institute on Alcohol Abuse and Alcoholism. The conference was designed to stimulate new approaches for understanding the effects of alcohol on behavior by bringing together researchers from two complementary fields: the experimental psychology of learning and memory and the investigation of alcohol and cognitive processes. Thus, on September 9th and 10th, 1976, a small group of researchers met in Laguna Beach, California, to share ideas about research on alcohol and memory, and to discuss the most promising directions for the expansion of knowledge about alcohol's influence on behavior.

Participants were invited to write about their current ideas on the study of human memory and, wherever possible, to tie these ideas to the study of alcohol's effects. The papers were circulated before the meeting and those that were presented at the conference and revised afterwards constitute the chapters of the present volume. These chapters offer a concise review of ongoing research and new directions in the study of alcohol and cognition. They will be of interest to students and researchers who are exploring the nature of cognitive deficits and the effects of alcohol on behavior, to clinicians in the area of alcoholism, and to members of the public and of governmental and private organizations who are interested in alcohol and behavior.

We wish to thank the National Institute on Alcohol Abuse and Alcoholism for sponsorship of the conference, and express our appreciation to the Director of the Institute, Dr. Ernest P. Noble, for his strong interest in the development of new directions in research. Dr. Albert Pawlowski, Chief of the Extramural Research Branch of the National Institute on Alcohol Abuse and Alcoholism, worked closely with us from the outset. His help has been invaluable, as has been the assistance provided by the University of California, Irvine, in preparing for the conference. We would also like to thank those who worked with us at various stages: Karen Anderson, Gillian Cannon, Joellen Hartley, Susan Solick, Ken Stern, and Sherry Tackett. And, finally, we are deeply grateful to all of the participants at the conference for making this important event such a resounding success.

I.M.B.
E.S.P.

**ALCOHOL AND
HUMAN MEMORY**

Part I

INTRODUCTION

1
Alcohol Research: New Directions

Elizabeth S. Parker

National Institute on Alcohol Abuse and Alcoholism

Isabel M. Birnbaum

University of California at Irvine

The chapters in this volume have been written by scientists who share a mutual concern with developing new directions for understanding alcohol's effects on the fundamental cognitive process of memory. In recent years, research on learning and research on alcohol have advanced at a rapid rate, albeit somewhat independently. In the area of verbal learning, sophisticated theories and procedures have been developed to explain the workings of normal memory processes. With increasing recognition of the seriousness of the alcohol abuse problem, more and more scientists have found themselves challenged by research in this area. The following chapters illustrate some of the substantial benefits that can result from the application of experimental methods in verbal learning to research on alcohol. A synthesis between these fields is a mutually beneficial process. It both improves the quality of alcohol research and provides a fertile testing ground for theories of human memory.

The effects of alcohol on the central nervous system are associated with a wide repertoire of behavioral alterations. Evidence has emerged implicating alcohol consumption in a variety of deficits in human memory. In the chapters that follow, a full spectrum of alcohol-related amnesias is covered, and new approaches are described for studying and understanding human memory. Some of the highlights of the chapters and relevance to alcohol research are outlined below.

Theories and methods developed in the field of verbal learning offer rich potential for application to the study of alcohol and memory. Some of the theories and methods already have been applied to studies of cognitive deficits; others undoubtedly will be used in the future. For example, what are the similarities between alcohol-induced deficits in memory and changes in memory that are seen with aging? Can similar theories or models of information processing be fruitfully applied to the analysis of these deficits? How have the severe memory deficits seen in Korsakoff patients been analyzed and further understood within a "levels of processing" framework? Why are differences in the rate of acquisition of new information by normal individuals often followed by identical rates of forgetting? Can the theories used to explain these facts also be used to understand the impairment of learning often seen with alcohol intoxication? Models of information processing are proposed that separate memory into different, perhaps overlapping, phases, and suggestions are made for ways in which to detect the stages of memory most influenced by alcohol intoxication. Recent research on the mutual influence of internal events and external events on the perceived frequency of these events is described, and the relevance of this work to alcohol research is discussed. Is the detection of recurrence information – a remarkably sensitive process in normal individuals – or the differentiation between thoughts and external events influenced by alcohol intoxication? Some of the seemingly inappropriate behaviors resulting from intoxication could very well be related to confusions between what *really* happened and what was imagined to have happened. Are memories for internally and externally generated events equally affected by alcohol, or is one more sensitive to the effects of intoxication than the other? These and similar questions are discussed in the chapters that follow, and a bridge is built between somewhat disparate areas of inquiry. Questions of methodology that arise in one field are applied to another. The critical importance of the selection of the dependent variable is discussed, for example, and it is shown that widely different conclusions might be drawn on the basis of apparently similar measures of behavior. In another vein, the alcoholic blackout is simulated in the laboratory, and an accidental procedural difference is shown to have a powerful effect on the phenomenon under investigation. These discussions bring methodological considerations into sharp focus and will inevitably increase the sophistication of methods used in future studies of cognitive impairment.

Probably the most common type of alcohol-related memory loss occurs during acute intoxication. Although this passes unnoticed in most drinkers, experimental studies have shown that even moderate doses of alcohol in social drinkers produce measurable decrements in memory and learning capacities. These studies are described in the chapters that follow. What types of models can explain these losses? Does alcohol affect consolidation of the trace? Storage of new information? Retrieval? Do memory losses in much simpler organisms than humans have implications for the explanation of deficits that are found in humans? Just how acute memory deficits are related to other behavioral effects of alcohol on anxiety, aggression, motivation, and the dynamics of interpersonal interaction are questions yet to be addressed by research in the area of alcohol and memory. Although losses in information-processing capacities cannot be expected to account for all of alcohol's acute effects, there is little doubt that decrements in this critical process have ramifications for other behavioral effects of alcohol. For example, is it possible that one of the rewarding aspects of drinking for certain people is an impairment in cognitive functioning? Might this impairment be related to a reduction in anxiety? As more refined approaches are used to study the effects of alcohol on memory, a greater clarification of alcohol's global effects is bound to come about. In addition, there is a real need to specify the effects of alcohol at the behavioral level so that the biological bases of those effects can be more fully explored.

Interest in the phenomenon of state-dependent learning has increased in recent years, and new approaches in verbal learning have been applied to a number of problems that arise in this area. It generally has been agreed that state-dependent learning can be viewed as a type of context-specific learning: optimum recall of learned information should depend upon reinstatement of the original learning conditions. Alcohol and other drugs may produce contextual changes by altering the subject's internal environment; these changes might lead to deficits when sober subjects try to recall information they learned while intoxicated or when intoxicated subjects try to recall information they learned in the sober state. The reasons for the frequent failure to find state dependency and the apparent unreliability of the phenomenon are discussed. Many questions are unanswered, whereas tentative answers have been given in some cases. Why is state dependency evident in some situations and not in others? Can state dependency be masked by other effects? What factors increase the likelihood that state dependency will be observed? Are specific conditions of storage or retrieval critical for the occurrence of state dependency? What are the implications of differences in degree of original learning in different states? State dependency is a particularly critical area of study, since there may be a relationship between the state-dependent effects of a drug and its abuse. It appears, for example, that drugs which produce state dependency also have a high liability of abuse. Whether this reflects the fact that both state dependency and abuse occur with centrally active drugs or whether there is a more direct causal relationship remains to be seen. The study of state dependency will be an area of major concern for years to come, and it is hoped that its coverage in this volume will increase not only the efficiency but also the value of future studies.

A number of memory disorders have been associated with the abuse of alcohol, among them the alcoholic blackout, disturbances in recent memory and abstracting ability in sober alcoholics, and the severe amnesia of Korsakoff's syndrome. The nature and extent of these deficits are explored in several chapters, and provocative questions are raised. The alcoholic blackout is discussed, and important questions are addressed. For example: Is the blackout a defect in registration? Is it reversible? Is the alcoholic blackout preventable? Studies of chronic alcoholics raise further questions: Is a measurable memory deficit characteristic of only a small subset of chronic alcoholics? Are memory deficits limited to the early, postwithdrawal stage? Do the deficits depend upon other factors in combination with the chronic use of alcohol? The generalization that long-term alcoholics exhibit memory deficits is questioned, and suggestions are made for future research. In another series of studies, patients with Korsakoff's syndrome served as subjects in the exploration of possible "processing" deficits in this syndrome. Here we see a theoretical framework that was developed to explain normal memory processes applied to increase our understanding of severe, chronic impairment of mnemonic functioning. Advances in research on cognitive deficits in alcoholic individuals will have beneficial spinoffs for understanding the development of alcoholism and for improving its treatment.

The preceding paragraphs serve merely to summarize some of the highlights of the conference on alcohol and human memory. No doubt the summary would be quite different if other participants were asked for their impressions. We found the conference to be a tremendously exciting and worthwhile experience, and our research has been substantially influenced by many of the issues brought out by the participants. We hope this volume will serve as a forum of ideas, questions, and directions for research on alcohol and memory. We look forward to an even greater collaboration between experimental psychologists in the area of learning and memory and investigators in the area of alcohol and behavior.

Part II

APPROACHES TO THE STUDY OF ALCOHOL AND MEMORY

2

Similarities Between the Effects of Aging and Alcoholic Intoxication on Memory Performance, Construed Within a "Levels of Processing" Framework

Fergus I. M. Craik

University of Toronto

Three related topics are treated in this chapter. First, theoretical and empirical work concerned with a "levels of processing" view of memory is briefly described. Second, some of the findings in the field of adult age differences in human memory are reviewed, since there appear to be strong parallels between the effects of aging and of alcohol intoxication on memory performance. An attempt is made to show how notions deriving from the levels of processing approach can provide a heuristic framework for the further exploration and fuller understanding of the effects of aging and of alcohol on memory. Finally, some speculations are advanced on the causes underlying the effects on memory of divided attention, aging, and alcoholic intoxication.

A "LEVELS OF PROCESSING" VIEW OF MEMORY

Craik and Lockhart (1972) put forward some arguments against the currently popular view that human memory could most usefully be viewed as a series of stages or stores. Instead, they suggested (following such attention theorists as Treisman, 1964, and Sutherland, 1968) that incoming stimuli are analyzed to different levels or depths, depending on such factors as the amenability of the stimulus to deep processing, the nature of the task, and the amounts of time and attention that the subject could devote to processing the items. In this context "depth" refers to a continuum of processing running from shallow sensory analyses requiring little attention to deeper semantic processes through which the stimulus is identified, interpreted, and enriched by associations with stored knowledge. Craik and Lockhart argued that the memory trace may be considered the record of those analyses performed during perception and comprehension of the stimulus and that deeper processing resulted in longer lasting traces. According to this view, both the qualitative nature of the trace and its persistence over time depend entirely on those cognitive operations performed during initial processing of the event. It is implicit in the argument that no further processes, such as consolidation, are necessary for the long-term registration of the memory trace.

Other points made by Craik and Lockhart include the acknowledgment that the distinction between short-term and long-term memory, in some form, is a necessary one. They suggested that items in "primary memory" (Waugh & Norman, 1965) are those phenomenologically "in mind"; such items reflect continued attention devoted to the active analysis of the event's mental representation. Once attention is diverted, information is lost from the trace at a rate that depends on its deepest level of analysis. Thus, short-term memory (or primary memory) is viewed as a *process* of continued activation rather than as a separate store. Finally, Craik and Lockhart urged that greater use be made of the incidental learning paradigm in memory research. The point here is that by specifying some operation to be performed on the item to be remembered, greater control is achieved over the subsequent mental operations than would be achieved by merely instructing subjects to "learn" or "remember" the item. The assumption is that real-life learning can be understood in terms of the mental operations performed during the learning period; further, that such operations can usefully be characterized as involving relatively shallow or deep levels of processing.

These notions were given some empirical substance by Craik and Tulving (1975). A typical experiment in this series involved presenting subjects with a different word on each of 60 trials. Before each word was presented, the subject was asked a question concerning either its structural characteristics (e.g., "Is the word in capital letters?"), its sound (e.g., "Does the word rhyme with DOOR?"), or its meaning (e.g., "Is the word a vegetable name?"). It was postulated that such questions necessitated progressively deeper analysis from structural to semantic questions and that a later memory test would thus show best retention of words associated with semantic questions and poorest retention of those associated with structural questions. This result was obtained in both recall and recognition and under both incidental and intentional learning instructions. Typical results are shown in Table 1. It also has been demonstrated that the superior retention of deeply processed words is not simply due to the longer

TABLE 1
Proportions of Words Recognized Under Various
Encoding Conditions[a]

	Question type		
	Case	Rhyme	Category
Positive responses	.23	.59	.81
Negative responses	.28	.33	.62

[a]From Craik & Tulving, 1975, Exp. 9. (Copyright 1975 by the American Psychological Association. Reprinted by Permission.)

decision times associated with semantic processing (Craik & Tulving, 1975); nor can the result be attributed to a failure to perceive the whole word in the shallow condition, since essentially the same pattern of results was obtained (a) when subjects wrote each word down at presentation and (b) the question was presented *after* the word was shown on each trial (Craik, 1977b).

One unexpected feature of the results shown in Table 1 is the generally poorer retention of words associated with negative responses (i.e., words that are *not* in capital letters, do *not* rhyme, or do *not* fit the category). Also, it has been found consistently that the retention difference between positive and negative responses is greatest for deeply processed items. To account for these findings, Craik and Tulving suggested that retention is enhanced by greater degrees of *elaboration* of the trace — that is, by an increase in the richness and complexity of the cognitive operations performed. In addition, they suggested that such elaboration was particularly likely to occur when the remembered item and its encoding context could be integrated to form a coherent unit. Positive responses in the Craik and Tulving paradigm represent instances where the item and its context (the encoding question) can be so integrated. That is, for positive responses, context and item together form a coherent elaborated trace, whereas for negative responses the potential for integration and elaboration is much less marked.

In one study (Craik & Tulving, 1975, Experiment 7) elaboration was directly manipulated by varying the complexity of a sentence frame with one word missing; the subject's task was to decide whether the word on each trial fitted into the frame on that trial. Figure 1 shows that in a later free-recall test, greater sentence complexity was associated with higher recall levels, but only for positive responses. Apparently, when the word and the sentence frame do not form a coherent unit (negative responses) the item does not benefit from greater trace elaboration. This pattern of results was amplified dramatically when the sentence frames were re-presented as cues. This manipulation had no effect on negative responses but boosted recall of positive responses, especially with more

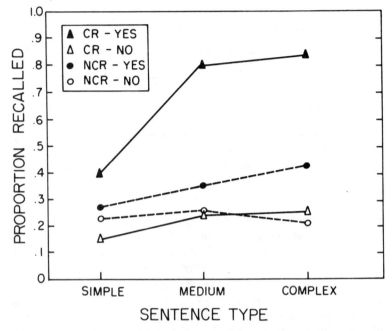

FIGURE 1   Proportion of words recalled as a function of sentence complexity. (Craik & Tulving, 1975, Exp. 7. Copyright 1975 by the American Psychological Association. Reprinted by permission.) CR = cued recall; NCR = noncued recall.

elaborate encodings. Thus, it may be concluded that for a retrieval cue to be effective, it must be present during encoding of the event and must also form an integral part of the item's functional encoding. Put another way, if the retrieval cue is successful in eliciting the item it may be inferred that the information in the cue is also contained in the item's encoded trace (Tulving & Thomson, 1973).

A further notion that we have been concerned with recently is the idea of *uniqueness* of memory traces. It seems possible that both increased "depth" and increased elaboration serve to make the trace more unique and thus more discriminable from other traces. Thus, it may be that shallow encodings are still present in the system but are so like thousands of encoded past events that they are not retrievable. Moscovitch and Craik (1976) found that when uniqueness was varied by having several items share the same encoding question retention levels of the items were lowered, and the encoding question was less effective as a retrieval cue. At the moment the notions of depth, elaboration, congruence of item and context, and uniqueness all seem to be important principles to further our understanding of memory processes.

One final theoretical point will be made in this context. It seems reasonable to argue that retrieval processes may be understood in exactly the same terms as encoding processes. That is, when a retrieval cue is presented, it is processed by the cognitive system in the same manner as the remembered item was processed originally. Again, the products of the cognitive analyses performed yield a particular percept. It may be postulated that "remembering" occurs when the same percepts are achieved at input and at retrieval. Thus, the notions of depth and elaboration may be used to describe retrieval processes as well as encoding processes.

To summarize these speculations (see also Lockhart, Craik & Jacoby, 1976) it is suggested that at input, an event is encoded in terms of the mental operations performed by the cognitive system during the processes of perception and comprehension. The nature of the encoding will be influenced both by the task presented to the subject and by the current state of the cognitive system; in turn, this state may be affected by a number of factors including expectations, set, context, age, fatigue, and drugs. These factors interact to yield an encoding of a certain uniqueness that incorporates various qualitative characteristics. Retrieval is successful to the extent that the information presented in the test phase can be processed by the cognitive system to yield a percept uniquely similar to the encoded percept. Thus retrieval will be enhanced as the retrieval information is made progressively more like the input information (including both the item and its context). Retrieval also will be enhanced to the extent that the cognitive system is in the same general state as it was at input (and is thus likely to treat the retrieval information in the same way as the input information was treated). Finally, retrieval will be enhanced to the extent that the encoded retrieval information uniquely specifies the sought-for item.

AGE DIFFERENCES IN MEMORY

Previous authors (Moskowitz & Burns, 1971; Ryback, 1971) have pointed out the parallels between the effects of aging and the effects of alcoholic intoxication on memory performance. In this section, some of these similarities will be described. The exact definition of "younger" and "older" differs from study to study, but typically the "young" subjects range in age from 18 to 30, whereas the "older" or "elderly" groups are made up of people aged between 60 and 80 years.

First, it is well established that age has a much larger detrimental effect on secondary memory performance. The terms primary memory (PM) and secondary memory (SM) are used in the sense described by Waugh and Norman (1965). Items in PM are those in mind, in conscious awareness; whereas SM items are those retrieved from "memory proper." The arguments for using PM and SM as the basic dichotomy in memory, rather than the confused and ill-specified terms, "immediate memory," "short-term" and "long-term memory," were provided initially by Waugh and Norman (1965) and are summarized by Craik and Levy

(1976). The essential argument is that whereas there do appear to be encoding, retention, and retrieval differences between items held in conscious awareness and those that must be retrieved from memory, there are no such *qualitative* differences between items retrieved from SM (in this sense) after 10 seconds and those retrieved after 10 hours. According to Waugh and Norman's analysis, the basic distinction is in terms of the different *processes* used, not in terms of time intervals. The PM/SM distinction has proved most useful in clarifying findings from studies using normal young adults as subjects, and it seems likely that this distinction also would play a useful role in disentangling the conclusions from "short-term memory" studies in which alcohol and alcoholics are involved.

In experiments where a list of unrelated words is given for free recall, it is typically found that recall of the last few words presented is at a particularly high level. This "recency effect" is commonly attributed to retrieval from PM, and it has been shown that this component of free recall performance is little affected by increasing age (Craik, 1968; Raymond, 1971). On the other hand, the same studies found marked age decrements in recall of words retrieved from earlier portions of the list — from SM by the present analysis. In the case of alcohol intoxication, the findings reported by Jones and Jones (this volume) show that intoxication impairs recall of early and middle, but not late, list items. In cases where the list of words is quite short (6 to 8 words, say), immediate recall will contain a large PM component, and losses due to age or to intoxication should be relatively slight; such findings have been reviewed by Craik (1977a) in the case of aging and reported by Weingartner and Murphy (this volume). Weingartner and Murphy's experiment also had a delayed recall condition in which recall of several lists was attempted after 20 minutes of a distracting activity. Such recall is, of course, from SM only, and substantial decrements due to intoxication were found. By the present analysis, memory span largely reflects PM recall, and in line with the argument above, only slight decrements in span have been reported for age differences (Craik, 1977a) and for the effects of alcohol (Ryback, 1971; Parker, Alkana, Birnbaum, Hartley & Noble, 1974).

Age decrements in PM functioning have been observed in certain circumstances, however. These include situations that demand the division of attention between two sources of information (Inglis & Caird, 1963), paradigms demanding the active reorganization of material held in PM (Broadbent & Gregory, 1965; Talland, 1965), and the Sternberg paradigm (Anders, Fozard & Lillyquist, 1972). To date, no systematic body of data relevant to these manipulations exists in the literature on alcoholic intoxication, but it has been found that the effects of alcohol are exacerbated under divided attention conditions (Moskowitz & Burns, 1971; Moskowitz & De Pry, 1968). Also, alcohol intake is associated with an increase in errors for PM items in the Sternberg paradigm (Tharp, Rundell, Lester & Williams, 1975).

A second set of findings relating the effects of aging and alcoholic intoxication have been reported by Wickelgren (1975a, 1975b). He presented a very long string of words to subjects; their task was to recognize repetitions of words in the string. Words were repeated at delays ranging from 2 min to 50 min. Recognition performance declined with increases in the retention interval, but the interesting finding was that age and alcohol were associated with decrements in the degree of initial learning. No differences in decay rates were observed between experimental and control groups in either case.

A third group of studies that, more speculatively, provides a parallel between the effects of aging and of alcohol concerns the beneficial effects of providing adequate cues at retrieval. Craik (1977a) has pointed out that elderly subjects appear to be at the greatest disadvantage relative to younger groups when the retrieval information is inadequate. Thus, elderly subjects show large decrements in noncued recall, but little if any decrement in cued recall (Laurence, 1967) or in recognition (Schonfield & Robertson, 1966; Warrington & Silberstein, 1970). Although this pattern of findings suggests a retrieval deficit in noncued recall, it is entirely possible that encoding deficits also occur in certain circumstances (Craik, 1977a). Is there evidence from the alcohol literature that memory losses are ameliorated when retrieval information is improved? Again no systematic studies exist yet, but there are suggestions that losses with recognition techniques are comparatively slight (Goodwin, Powell, Bremer, Hoine & Stern, 1969; Wickelgren, 1975b). With regard to cued recall, Weiskrantz and Warrington (1970) have reported an attenuation of the memory loss exhibited by Korsakoff patients when a "partial cuing" technique was used. Also, Eich, Weingartner, Stillman, and Gillin (1975) demonstrated the beneficial effects of cues under marijuana intoxication. Thus, there are indirect indications that memory losses under alcoholic intoxication may also be ameliorated by the provision of adequate retrieval information.

The final area of similarity between the effects of aging and of alcoholic intoxication concerns the notion of levels of processing discussed earlier. Sharon White conducted a study (reported by Craik, 1977a) to test the notion that older subjects were capable of carrying out deep semantic encoding, which would support good memory performance, but that they did not spontaneously generate such encodings. She presented single words to young and old subjects under four encoding conditions: (1) capital letters; (2) rhyme; (3) category; and (4) "learn this word." The subjects expected a memory test for the "learn" words but thought they were merely making perceptual judgments in the other three conditions. After the encoding phase, subjects were given a free-recall test for all words, followed by a recognition test. Results are shown in Figure 2. Recall levels increased from "capitals" to category judgments; the "learn" words yielded retention levels equivalent to the semantic (category) task. Age decrements were found under three of the four conditions. This result was interpreted to mean that even when encoding was equated between young and older subjects, an age decrement remained due to less effective retrieval operations in the elderly. When retrieval, too, was constrained by the provision of more adequate retrieval information in recognition, age differences disappeared in all

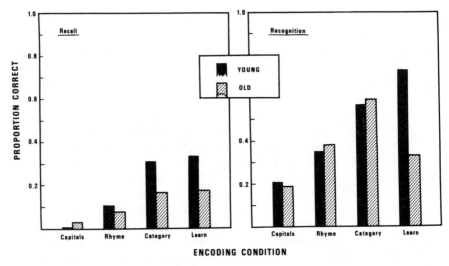

FIGURE 2   Age differences in recall and recognition as a function of level of processing (Craik, 1977a).

three incidental conditions. The observation that an age decrement remained in the "learn" condition may reflect less adequate encoding by the elderly group in that case. Similar patterns of results also have been reported by Lauer (1975) and by Eysenck (1974). The conclusion is that older subjects carry out fewer spontaneous encoding operations — especially those of a deep or elaborate nature — at both input and retrieval of remembered events.

A rather direct demonstration of this postulate was provided by Hulicka and Grossman (1967). When no mediators were provided in a paired associate learning task older subjects performed very poorly (13% recall as opposed to 63% recalled by a young group); when mediators were provided both age groups improved, but the older subjects benefited more — recall levels were now 65% and 83% for old and young subjects respectively. Again the conclusion was that older subjects are capable of using deeper semantic information but failed to generate it spontaneously. In the phrase of developmental psychologists, they exhibit a "production deficiency."

It is tempting to speculate that the memory deficits observed with the acute and chronic effects of alcohol can also be attributed to a failure to process deeply. This is the position argued by Cermak and Butters (1973) and by Cermak (this volume). The clustering deficit under alcohol intoxication reported by Parker et al. (1974) also may be described as a failure to involve deeper cognitive structures. Also, there is some evidence that memory deficits with alcohol are less severe when good retrieval information is provided; that is, when the subject is less reliant on spontaneous reconstructive activities as in recognition as opposed to recall (Goodwin et al., 1969).

Finally, if the effects of alcohol intoxication are similar to those of aging, in some respects at least, it would be predicted that no memory deficits would occur in intoxicated subjects if they were given orienting tasks to perform on words to be remembered (rather than simply being told to learn them) and if they were tested by recognition (Figure 2). In a very informal pilot study, I have found that mildly intoxicated subjects achieved normal scores on the levels of processing paradigm described above (Table 1). Clearly, however, this study has to be performed under properly controlled conditions. It is predicted that greater memory decrements due to alcohol intoxication should be observed under the "learn this word" condition than under orienting task conditions. Also, decrements would be expected to occur with larger doses of alcohol (especially where retention is assessed by recall), as performance on the orienting task would eventually suffer and encoding would be less adequate. An experiment yielding this pattern of results has been conducted recently by Isabel Birnbaum (personal communication).

UNDERLYING CAUSES

In the previous section it was argued that the effects of aging on memory are similar to those of alcohol intoxication. It was suggested that both deficits may be viewed as failures of the cognitive system to process information to sufficient depth, or with sufficient elaboration. What lies behind this processing failure? Why might it take more effort for an older person or an intoxicated person to achieve the performance levels of a young, sober subject?

A tentative answer is that both aging and intoxication result in a reduction of available processing resources. In the case of alcoholic intoxication, the idea of a reduction in either the amount or the rate of information processing has been extensively explored and supported by Burns, Moskowitz, and their colleagues (Burns, 1972; Moskowitz & Burns, 1971, 1976; Moskowitz & Roth, 1971; Moskowitz & Sharma, 1974) and by Hamilton and Copeman (1970). The notion is given added credibility by the results of an ongoing series of experiments by Dr. Alan Allport of Reading University, England. In outline, Allport has found that divided attention situations (which may be thought of as reducing available processing capacity) give rise to memory deficits that mimic the effects of some clinical amnesias. In one such experiment, Allport tested two groups of subjects — one under divided attention conditions (DA) and one control group (C). All subjects were given two lists of words to learn; one list was presented in the kitchen of their student apartment, and the other list was presented in the bedroom. The C group simply attempted to learn the words, whereas the DA group performed a concurrent arithmetic task while learning the words. In a recognition test 24 hours later, both groups scored quite highly (C = 98.8%; DA = 89.2%). When subjects then were asked to indicate whether each recognized word had been learned in the kitchen or in the bedroom, however, C subjects were able to do this with high accuracy (95.3%), whereas DA subjects responded at a chance level (46.2%). Whereas both groups apparently achieved a reasonable basic encoding of the words, only the undivided attention subjects had sufficient capacity to also encode peripheral details of the context with each word.

I should stress that Dr. Allport's description of his results is somewhat different from the account given above. He sees the "limited capacity" interpretation as rather too diffuse in that it does not specify the type of processing restricted. Following Huppert and Piercy (1976), Allport views his results as demonstrating a specific failure to integrate items with their temporal/spatial context under conditions of divided attention.

If the effects of aging resemble the effects of alcoholic intoxication and both are mimicked by learning under divided attention conditions (D. A. Allport, personal communication), it is reasonable to suppose that a *combination* of these factors would be particularly disastrous for memory functioning. There is good evidence that this is the case. It is well established that the effects of aging on memory are exacerbated under such DA conditions as dichotic listening (see Craik, 1977a). It also has been suggested (Parsons & Prigatano, this volume) "that alcoholism may interact with age so that the older the alcoholic, the more severe the intellectual deficit [p. 186]." Ryback (1971) tentatively proposed that "alcohol compounds the insult to the ongoing 'natural' progressive degeneration of a person's capacity for short-term memory that occurs with age [p. 1008]." In support of this conclusion, Cermak and Ryback (1976) have reported that age exacerbates the effects of alcohol on a short-term memory task.

Are the detrimental effects of alcoholic intoxication on memory exacerbated under conditions of divided attention? Studies by Burns (1972) and by Moskowitz and De Pry (1968) suggest an affirmative answer to this question. As a final piece of evidence, I will conclude with an account of a recent informal study by Eileen Simon and me that further suggests such an interaction. The experiment was first run on "normal" subjects (i.e., young, sober subjects) to test whether deeper processing consumes more processing capacity. The subjects monitored a visually presented series of words for the presence of targets defined either structurally, phonemically, or semantically; at the same time they performed an auditory digit–probe memory task. For the present purposes the normal group tested under semantic monitoring conditions will be compared with a group of similar subjects who had been drinking. After performing the divided attention task all subjects were given a recognition test for some of the visually presented words – both "targets" (i.e., words that did fit the monitored category) and nontargets. The results (Table 2) show that the drinking group performed as well as the controls on the initial tasks but less well on the subsequent recognition test. Although the effects are not large, 8 out of the 11 drinking subjects were below the mean for normals on recognition of nontargets; and all 11 were below the normal mean for targets. Again this is an experiment that must be run with

TABLE 2
Proportions Correct in a Divided-Attention Task and in a Subsequent Recognition Test
(Simon & Craik, Unpublished Study).

	Divided attention		Recognition	
	Probe-digit	Word detection	Targets	Nontargets
Sober subjects	.58	.93	.94	.46
Drinking subjects	.63	.92	.84	.41

proper controls; however, it is an interesting speculation that drinking subjects were able to perform the initial task but only at the cost of attenuating the normally occurring elaboration of the visually presented words. That is, they processed the words sufficiently to identify their category but not sufficiently to support good recognition in the subsequent, unexpected retention test.

SUMMARY

In summary, it has been suggested that the deleterious effects of alcoholic intoxication bear some striking resemblances to the effects of aging on memory performance. Both sets of effects may be due to a curtailment of the "elaborate," "deep," or "extensive" processing of events that occurs in the normal cognitive system and that supports later memory for those events. It was further suggested that this hypothesized curtailment of processing is due to a reduction in processing resources similar to that found under divided attention conditions. Further work will attempt to obtain sounder empirical support for the present suggestions and will examine the adequacy of the levels of processing framework to provide a fuller understanding of the effects observed.

ACKNOWLEDGMENTS

The empirical work reported was supported by grant A8261 from the National Research Council of Canada. The author gratefully acknowledges the help of Drs. D. A. Allport and L. L. Jacoby in developing the theoretical ideas.

REFERENCES

Anders, T. R., Fozard, J. L., & Lillyquist, T. D. The effects of age upon retrieval from short-term memory. *Developmental Psychology*, 1972, 6, 214–217.
Broadbent, D. E., & Gregory, M. Some confirmatory results on age differences in memory for simultaneous stimulation. *British Journal of Psychology*, 1965, 56, 77–80.

Burns, M. M. A test of information processing limits: Interactions of information load, alcohol effects, and age effects. Unpublished PhD dissertation, University of California, Irvine, 1972.

Cermak, L. S., & Butters, N. Information processing deficits of alcoholic Korsakoff patients. *Quarterly Journal of Studies on Alcohol,* 1973, *34,* 1110–1132.

Cermak, L. S., & Ryback, R. S. Recovery of verbal short-term memory in alcoholics. *Journal of Studies in Alcohol,* 1976, *37,* 46–52.

Craik, F. I. M. Two components in free recall. *Journal of Verbal Learning and Verbal Behavior,* 1968, *7,* 996–1004.

Craik, F. I. M. Age differences in human memory. In J. E. Birren and K. W. Schaie (Eds.), *Handbook of the psychology of aging.* New York: Van Nostrand Reinhold, 1977. (a)

Craik, F. I. M. Depth of processing in recall and recognition. In S. Dornic (Ed.), *Attention and performance VI.* Hillsdale, N.J.: Lawrence Erlbaum Associates, 1977. (b)

Craik, F. I. M., & Levy, B. A. The concept of primary memory. In W. K. Estes (Ed.), *Handbook of learning and cognitive processes. Vol. 4: Attention and Memory.* Hillsdale, N.J.: Lawrence Erlbaum Associates, 1976.

Craik, F. I. M., & Lockhart, R. S. Levels of processing: A framework for memory research. *Journal of Verbal Learning and Verbal Behavior,* 1972, *11,* 671–684.

Craik, F. I. M., & Tulving, E. Depth of processing and the retention of words in episodic memory. *Journal of Experimental Psychology: General,* 1975, *104,* 268–294.

Eich, J. E. Weingartner, H., Stillman, R. C., & Gillin, J. C. State-dependent accessibility of retrieval cues in the retention of a categorized list. *Journal of Verbal Learning and Verbal Behavior,* 1975, *14,* 408–417.

Eysenck, M. W. Age differences in incidental learning. *Developmental Psychology,* 1974, *10,* 936–941.

Goodwin, D. W., Powell, B., Bremer, D., Hoine, H., & Stern, J. Alcohol and recall: State dependent effects in man. *Science,* 1969, *163,* 1358–1360.

Hamilton, P. & Copeman, A. The effect of alcohol and noise on components of a tracking and monitoring task. *British Journal of Psychology,* 1970, *61,* 149–156.

Hulicka, I. M., & Grossman, J. Age-group comparisons for the use of mediators in paired-associate learning. *Journal of Gerontology,* 1967, *22,* 46–51.

Huppert, F. A., & Piercy, M. Recognition memory in amnesic patients: Effect of temporal context and familiarity of material. *Cortex,* 1976, *12,* 3–20.

Inglis, J., & Caird, W. K. Age differences in successive responses to simultaneous stimulation. *Canadian Journal of Psychology,* 1963, *17,* 98–105.

Lauer, P. A. The effects of different types of word processing on memory performance in young and elderly adults. Unpublished PhD thesis, University of Colorado, 1975.

Laurence, M. W. Memory loss with age: A test of two strategies for its retardation. *Psychonomic Science,* 1967, *9,* 209–210.

Lockhart, R. S., Craik, F. I. M., & Jacoby, L. Depth of processing, recognition and recall. In J. Brown (Ed.), *Recall and recognition.* London: Wiley, 1976.

Moscovitch, M., & Craik, F. I. M. Depth of processing, retrieval cues, and uniqueness of encoding as factors in recall. *Journal of Verbal Learning and Verbal Behavior,* 1976, *15,* 447–458.

Moskowitz, H., & Burns, M. Effect of alcohol on the psychological refractory period. *Quarterly Journal of Studies on Alcohol,* 1971, *32,* 782–790.

Moskowitz, H., & Burns, M. Effects of rate of drinking on human performance. *Journal of Studies on Alcohol,* 1976, *37,* 598–605.

Moskowitz, H., & De Pry, D. Differential effect of alcohol on auditory vigilance and divided-attention tasks. *Quarterly Journal of Studies on Alcohol,* 1968, *29,* 54–63.

Moskowitz, H., & Roth, S. Effect of alcohol on response latency in object naming. *Quarterly Journal of Studies on Alcohol,* 1971, *32,* 969–975.

Moskowitz, H., & Sharma, S. Effects of alcohol on peripheral vision as a function of attention. *Human Factors,* 1974, *16,* 174–180.

Parker, E. S., Alkana, R. L., Birnbaum, I. M., Hartley, J. T., & Noble, E. P. Alcohol and the disruption of cognitive processes. *Archives of General Psychiatry,* 1974, *31,* 824–828.

Raymond, B. J. Free recall among the aged. *Psychological Reports,* 1971, *29,* 1179–1182.

Ryback, R. S. The continuum and specificity of the effects of alcohol on memory. A review. *Quarterly Journal of Studies on Alcohol,* 1971, *32,* 995–1016.

Schonfield, D., & Robertson, B. A. Memory storage and aging. *Canadian Journal of Psychology,* 1966, *20,* 228–236.

Sutherland, N. S. Outlines of a theory of visual pattern recognition in animals and man. *Proceedings of the Royal Society, Series B.,* 1968, *171,* 297–317.

Talland, G. A. Three estimates of the word span and their stability over the adult years. *Quarterly Journal of Experimental Psychology,* 1965, *17,* 301–307.

Tharp, V. K., Jr., Rundell, O. H., Jr., Lester, B. K., & Williams, H. L. Alcohol and secobarbital: Effects on information processing. In M. M. Gross (Ed.), *Alcohol intoxication and withdrawal: Experimental Studies II.* New York: Plenum Press, 1975.

Treisman, A. Monitoring and storage of irrelevant messages in selective attention. *Journal of Verbal Learning and Verbal Behavior,* 1964, *3,* 449–459.

Tulving, E., & Thomson, D. M. Encoding specificity and retrieval processes in episodic memory. *Psychological Review,* 1973, *80,* 352–373.

Warrington, E. K., & Silberstein, M. A. A questionnaire technique for investigating very long-term memory. *Quarterly Journal of Experimental Psychology,* 1970, *22,* 508–512.

Waugh, N. C., & Norman, D. A. Primary memory. *Psychological Review,* 1965, *72,* 89–104.

Weiskrantz, L., & Warrington, E. K. A study of forgetting in amnesic patients. *Neuropsychologia,* 1970, *8,* 281–288.

Wickelgren, W. A. Age and storage dynamics in continuous recognition memory. *Developmental Psychology,* 1975, *11,* 165–169. (a)

Wickelgren, W. A. Alcoholic intoxication and memory storage dynamics. *Memory and Cognition,* 1975, *3,* 385–389. (b)

3

Remarks on the Detection and Analysis of Memory Deficits

Thomas K. Landauer

Bell Laboratories, Murray Hill, New Jersey

It has been long and widely suspected, and heterogeneously demonstrated by clinical and experimental evidence, that alcoholic intoxication has a detrimental effect on memory. Cultural wisdom has it that there is a variety of different effects: general befuddlement while intoxicated, the occasional "blackout" afterward, and progressive deterioration with long-term use. If there is even some truth in this knowledge, there is an enormous practical issue involved and a striking opportunity to gain fundamental knowledge about mental mechanisms.

Laboratory experimentation on memory has been going on for about 100 years now; it would seem that the tools for exploring such problems should be at hand. Despite this, intensive experimental study of alcohol and memory seems to have just begun. I think this reflects an unfortunate failure in the development of the psychology of learning, a failure to learn sufficiently from pathology. The means by which learning deficits are clinically detected, monitored, and analyzed are not always the same and do not always reflect the same variables as do contemporary laboratory paradigms for studying the conditions and processes of human learning. For example, clinical usage sometimes defines "immediate memory" rather vaguely as "immediately after the learning experience," short-term memory as that remaining about a half-hour later, and long-term memory as recollection after a day or more. By contrast, current wisdom in experimental psychology usually distinguishes sensory storage of about a second, a subsequent "short-term" or "active memory" with storage times measured in seconds or minutes (or 5 to 10 intervening items), and "long-term" storage that is sometimes assumed to be measurable as little as a half-minute later. Although there is considerable confusion in the temporal definitions of the various theoretically posited "stores," the modal durations for what experimental psychologists tend to view as "short-term" and "long-term" processes are one to two orders of magnitude shorter than those sometimes used by clinicians.

Whether such differences reflect genuine differences in evidence or are simply due to inadequacies in communication between the two camps, it would seem a useful exercise to discuss how current experimentalists would subdivide the important phases and processes of memory and how they would propose to differentially measure effects on them.

OUTLINE OF TEMPORAL ORGANIZATION OF INFORMATION PROCESSING IN HUMAN MEMORY

In recent years several memory researchers have outlined such schemes (Atkinson & Shiffrin, 1968; Sperling, 1967; Waugh & Norman, 1965; Wickelgren, 1974). Although the differences themselves may be interesting (as a rough measure of our reliability, if nothing else), it is not my intention here to review this work; good reviews exist (e.g., Baddeley, 1976; Crowder, 1976). The time chart in Figure 1 gives an approximation to my own current view of the matter. My plan is to outline this view briefly and to discuss in detail some of its less familiar aspects. The time chart diagrams various processes to which information is subjected as it is collected, stored, and used. I will begin at the top and proceed downward, discussing each phase, then go back and suggest methods by which deficiencies in each phase might be differentially diagnosed.

Initial Registration and Interpretation

The first proposed stage of memory processing is initial registration. It consists of apprehension of sensory data. It is modulated by an attentive gate. By this I mean such mundane factors as whether one is looking out the window when a visual stimulus is presented and also less observable conditions as whether one is asleep or engaged in a distracting fantasy. After registration, there is interpretation. For example when a subject is shown a word to remember, he must translate the pattern of visual edges and light areas into a "word." There is evidence that one does recall the details of typography, place on the page, and so forth, (e.g., Rothkopf, 1971); however, we do primarily recall words as words, and words are not words until an act of interpretation has been performed. This interpretation always depends on the application of prior knowledge about the presented object and usually takes the form of a classification of the object — e.g., as an exemplar or token of the word *horse*.

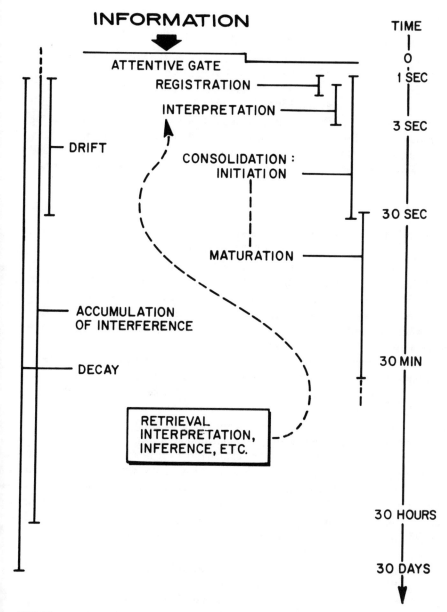

FIGURE 1 Schematic time chart showing postulated storage (on the right) and loss (on the left) processes in the information flow of memory. The indicated times are approximate modal half-life durations for the processes.

Consolidation

Following interpretation, or perhaps overlapping it, there is a process that I have labeled "consolidation." By this I mean something much more general than what is sometimes meant in physiological circles. Any process that makes the received input less subject to forgetting, more likely to be remembered later, is included. This does not mean only biochemically or neurologically defined events but also admits "cognitive" work. Consolidation is subdivided into two components. One is *initiation* — setting the process in motion — the other *maturation* — actually accomplishing it. One of the points I discuss in detail involves consolidation and consideration of this distinction, so I will postpone elaboration of these issues.

Loss Processes

The time chart also shows three processes that tend to cause losses at different rates. First is a process labeled "drift." This is a representation or abstraction of the often observed fact that things learned very recently are remembered better than things learned less recently, and that as time passes the confusion between things learned earlier and things learned later increases primarily to the detriment of the more recently learned material. This process is perhaps best exemplified in the rapid loss — over 30 seconds or so — of the ability to reproduce a small set of symbols, as measured by the Brown—Peterson—Peterson paradigm in which recall is probed after varying amounts of interfering activity. The rate of loss of memory in this situation is highly sensitive to the amount of potentially confusing information that has been learned just previously. This phase is also associated with the rapid change in memory for the last 5 to 10 items in a series, which for a brief period enjoy an advantage over previously presented items, then merge with them in likelihood of recollection.

There are currently many competing explanations for this phase of rapid initial forgetting in the presence of interference. I have purposely chosen the term "drift" both to prevent identification of this phase exclusively with any one of the current theoretical interpretations of it and to suggest its possible relation to the notions of contextual drift proposed by Bower (1972), the stimulus sampling fluctuation of Estes (1955), and the random walk through memory posited by Landauer (1975). All of these, in different ways, explain the initial rapid loss as a part of a single forgetting process rather than a manifestation of a separate "short-term" store. I do this not because I am sure there is no separate short-term store but because I think that this analysis of the phenomenon may be less familiar to workers outside the field of memory, and because it suggests different means of exploring memorial effects. Thus, another topic to be discussed in greater depth comes from an elaboration of this analysis.

The second source of retention decrement is the continued addition to memory of new material that may be difficult to discriminate from what was learned before and therefore make differential retrieval more difficult. The third factor is passive decay or loss. (I realize that there is considerable debate and strong opinion as to whether this occurs, but I know of no data that definitively settle the issue.)

Retrieval

Finally, the time chart shows a process of retrieval. This refers to how the information previously stored in memory is gotten back, separated from other potentially confusing material, reconstructed, and added to by inference from other information in memory. There is a dotted arrow leading back from the retrieval processes to the interpretive phase to indicate that retrieval of information stored earlier is a necessary part of interpretation. Similarly, the interpretation of a question or cue and of the stored information is a necessary part of retrieval. Methods for the study of retrieval are relatively new, so I will also give them special attention.

Single-Store Representation of Memory

Let me dwell a bit here on the absence in Figure 1 of separate short- and long-term memories and connections between them. By this abstention I do not mean to claim that no such things exist, only that most known properties of the dynamics of information flow in and out of memory can be represented in other ways.[1] At least two recent theories of memory that assume only one form of storage provide excellent quantitative accounts of the major temporal functions in forgetting, as well as many of the other facts that usually are taken as evidence of dual storage. One (Wickelgren, 1974) is an updated, sophisticated strength model with two trace properties, both of which are subject to change but at different rates. The other (Landauer, 1975) is a random storage model in which drift in the region of memory being used gives rise to temporal properties. The latter provides an analysis that may be of special interest in the context of alcohol research. One of the most compelling arguments for the dual store idea is the existence of clinical memory pathologies in which memories of different ages appear to be differentially impaired. Indeed, Wickelgren (1968) wrote, "what is overwhelmingly supported by . . . the studies of H. M. and subjects with similar deficits, is that there are at least two different memory traces in normal subjects, a short-term trace and a long-term trace [p. 242]."

[1] The major exceptions involve what Sternberg (1966) has called "active memory." The retrieval and transformation of information from newly learned short lists of items manifest properties that have not yet been explained adequately without postulating a special state. For completeness, Figure 1 might well include a "box" representing active or working memory. It would be located in approximately the same time region as registration and interpretation.

However, the random storage theory, which hypothesizes only one memory store and has only one parameter related directly to the rate of forgetting, could give rise to memory disorders that resemble closely the clinical syndromes that are taken as evidence of dual storage. Let me sketch the relevant aspects of the theory. Memory is represented as a large, three-dimensional array of general purpose data registers. At any point in time, one and only one register is available for data entry. A fairly large number of registers in the region surrounding this central register — but not the entire memory — can be interrogated for previously stored information. The location of the active zone drifts slowly and randomly. Thus, each new datum is stored in a register whose location is determined only by chance temporal drift. Similarly, the part of memory from which data can be drawn at any one time is determined only by the same random drift. There is multiple copy storage of information that is encountered repeatedly. Each time a fact — old or new — is stored, it is stored in the currently available register. Thus, facts encountered many times will be stored in many places. If many experiences with the same fact are well distributed in time, their storage loci will tend to be well distributed in memory. At retrieval, only data from a limited region surrounding the entry register can be reached. Therefore, a particular fact will, on average, be found with greater certainty and less search time the more often, the more widely distributed, and the more recently it has been stored.

A wide variety of known phenomena are exhibited by this very simple mechanism including: classic learning curves, forgetting curves with realistic complex shapes, several gross and subtle spacing phenomena, frequency and recency effects on retrieval time, associative facilitation effects, and several more. Many more complex cognitive phenomena do not follow directly from the theory but can be explained by using the memory as a component of a larger overall processing system. For more details, see Landauer (1975).

Several contrasting syndromes of memory deficit could occur as a result of malfunctions of mechanisms postulated by this theory. Here is a sample. First, suppose the drift of the active region ceased or slowed down greatly. New data would always be entered in the same registers, overwriting what was there before. There would be good recollection of the last stored event. There also would be normal retrieval of information stored in the region accessible to interrogation. Since this region would contain a random sample of previously stored information, it would be relatively certain to contain at least one record of familiar, well-rehearsed facts. Thus, "old" memories would appear largely unaffected. But, because of constant overwriting, the storage of new, permanent memories would be greatly impeded.

Second, suppose the drift became extremely rapid. There would not be overwriting, and entry of new data with repeated study would be normal or even better. But because the active region would drift away so fast "short-term" memory for a singly presented item would be subject to abnormally rapid decline.

Third, suppose that the active region was made to shift suddenly from one place to another. Information acquired just before the shift would appear to be lost, because the registers in which it was stored could no longer be reached for interrogation. But old, multiply stored information still would be retrievable. The greater the shift, the larger, on the average, would be the temporal extent of this retrograde amnesia, because (due to the slow random drift) nearness in memory reflects nearness in time of receipt. Moreover, unless the sudden shift was caused by an irreversible aversion to a particular region of memory, the lost memories would tend to be regained as drift brought the active region back to where it was when the shift occurred. On the average, older memories — those stored farther from the location at the time of shift — would be recovered first.

These three kinds of hypothetical malfunctions resemble, respectively, the classic temporal lobe syndrome described by Milner (1966), the syndrome described by Shallice and Warrington (1970) and the syndrome of posttraumatic retrograde amnesia. Although they may not account for all aspects of the clinical pathologies, they do mimic almost perfectly those features of memory disorders that are often thought to require a dual store explanation. Let me stress one logical point. Even if the random storage model is not correct, it nevertheless constitutes a clear proof by counterexample that differential impairment of old and new memories does not imply the existence of two separate stores.

Just to round out this digression, let me note that the random store model suggests still other hypothetical memory dysfunctions. For one, suppose the slowdown of drift discussed first were only partial. Learning would occur but with extra difficulty because of frequent overwriting. Interference effects would be magnified relative to the normal, because information received in a limited time period would tend to be stored more densely and consequently retrieved less independently. Added discrimination cues and greater temporal separation of presentation of potentially interfering materials would be especially helpful to people with such a dysfunction. For another possibility, suppose the region accessible to interrogation shrank. All memories would be preserved, but fewer could be retrieved at any one moment. Memory would be subject to abnormally large fluctuation. Either this malfunction or the extra-rapid drift possibility, discussed second above, would make a person's mind "seem to wander." Finally, suppose the data entry mechanism became erratic. Initial storage functions would be impaired; but once learned, information would be retained normally. But more interestingly, people with such a disorder would learn as if they were being given fewer, but more widely spaced trials, compared to normals. There is no reason to believe that a particular patient would be subject to only one such symptom; instead, one might expect some physiological disturbances to produce multiple malfunctions.

DURATION OF PHASES

The righthand side of Figure 1 contains an approximate time line (distorted) to indicate when and for how long these various phases and processes occur.

In most cases the durations of these processes appear to be something like negative-exponentially distributed, so that their durations might best be described by half lives or medians. The times are both inexact and intrinsically variable for several reasons; for one, the durations involved are not all definable purely as a function of time. Often they are critically influenced by what fills the time. Thus the values shown are intended to suggest the probable modal values under ecologically representative conditions, rather than minimum or maximum values.

Registration and Interpretation

The period for registration is estimated from the times that a visual stimulus needs to be available in order to be recognized (Sperling, 1960). The time for interpretive processes is a rough guess, based on the time subjects usually spend answering easy questions about such items as those they are asked to remember in learning experiments. For example, people spend about 1 second deciding whether a word is the name of a fish or of a living thing with wings. When asked to retrieve previously learned word associates, they usually give correct answers within 3 or 4 seconds. Presuming that a similar classification or inference is made in the interpretive phase of storage of new information, 1 second or 2 probably should suffice.

Consolidation

Consolidation initiation refers to the process by which an experience induces the system to store information. The duration of the phase in which this occurs is based on experiments in which interference by potentially confusing items was used to disrupt the formation of memory for a previously presented item. The interval over which disruption can be obtained provides a lower bound on the duration of the consolidation period. Consolidation could be going on even when it is not possible to interfere with it in this way, but it must be going on at times when such time-dependent disruption can occur. I have, arbitrarily for now, associated the initiation phase of consolidation with the period over which input events can be especially disruptive. The suggested length of this phase also corresponds to the period over which variations in spacing between two presentations are effective in modulating later recall. I argue below that it is reasonable to attribute such variations to factors associated with consolidation.

It also has been found (e.g., Landauer, 1974) that the effects of such psychological anticonsolidation manipulations as these are not felt immediately. If one tests too soon there is no benefit attributable to postponement of interfering material (or to postponement of the repetition of an item). On the other hand, if one waits 20 minutes there are big effects. This and other consolidation phenomena are discussed in more detail below. For now, the time for *maturation* of consolidation shown in Figure 1 is meant to approximate the period over which these effects become manifest.

Loss Processes

Among the information loss factors, drift happens over a half life of about 30 seconds, an estimate from Brown–Peterson–Peterson type distractor–probe experiments or intralist tests (e.g., Landauer, 1969). The build-up of retroactive interference and passive decay seem to be continuous processes that go on for life.

Retrieval events happen in the same sort of time spans as do entry and interpretation events, that is, in a matter of seconds.

EXPERIMENTAL METHODS FOR
DIFFERENTIAL DIAGNOSES

A brief outline of the kinds of experimental tasks that can be used to measure the various assumed processes follows, with particular attention to methods that might be suitable for alcohol research. Two main matters — consolidation and retrieval dynamics — are emphasized, because they have not received sufficiently careful analysis in this context.

General Experimental Approaches

First, let us review some of the ways experimental observations can be used to determine the locus of effects of known memory-altering factors. At the most general level, there are two means available for isolating the locus of a memorial effect. The first approach requires knowledge of *when* a particular phase occurs, so that a drug can be made present only at that time. Figure 1 provides an analysis that will support this approach. The second approach is to make measurements that are sensitive only to impairments of a particular process.

Registration and Interpretation

Now let us start at the top of the set of processes shown in Figure 1 and briefly outline methods that might be used to tap each of them. Since registration and interpretation are at the front end of the information stream, one might be tempted to try to study them by the "method of deletion." One would try to tap their output before other factors need be applied. For example, the experimenter might ask for speeded recognition of well-known words with and without alcohol. But that wouldn't work, because a person can't indicate even that registration has occurred without some response and all the rest of the information processing that a response entails.

Perhaps a better method would be to apply the additive factors reaction-time method developed by Sternberg (see e.g., 1969 a, b). In this approach one would make the registration or interpretation more or less difficult, perhaps by degrading the physical stimulus representing the information to be stored. If the time required to respond to the stimulus were more (or less) influenced by degradation with alcohol than without it, one could conclude that alcohol affects the same process as does degradation.

Let us consider the interpretation process further. Perhaps the nicest way of demonstrating the influence of selective interpretive activity on learning is Gieselman's (1975) recent variation on Bjork's directed forgetting paradigm. In Geiselman's task a subject is given a long passage to read that contains — among other things — information about two different topics, for example Jefferson and Washington. The subject is instructed to forget information pertaining to one of the two topics, say Washington. Compared to noninstructed controls, those instructed to forget about Washington remember more about Jefferson. Crossing this experiment factorially with variations in drugs would tell us whether the drug debilitates a person in the use of this memory device. (But see remarks below on pitfalls in such interactive designs when the response measure is probability correct rather than reaction time.)

Two-Stage Consolidation

Consolidation is a particularly interesting and perhaps particularly difficult case. It is particularly interesting because one could suspect that a depressant drug like alcohol would have an anticonsolidating effect by analogy with results observed in laboratory animals with similar acting drugs. One problem is that the time course of consolidation in human learning is not known. From retrograde interference experiments it appears to be rather brief, whereas the onset time of alcohol effect is rather long. If human consolidation were limited to the rather brief period during which retrograde interference works, the traditional laboratory demonstrations of time-dependent, posttrial drug effects would be very difficult to perform. However, as already mentioned, it is possible to believe that there is a second phase of consolidation that is probably longer and therefore more promising as a target for drug research.

Let me briefly review the relevant work on consolidation in human paired-associate learning that we have conducted. The basic experimental paradigm is as follows. The subject is shown a series of paired associates consisting of three-letter nonsense syllables and digits. Each pair appears once and only once, for 10 seconds; and there are about 30 of them. Then there is a 20- to 30-minute rest interval occupied by some distracting activity and finally, a test in which the subjects attempt to recall the digits that appeared with each nonsense syllable. Figure 2 schematizes a typical experiment. The first pair presented is a buffer; then there are two "critical" items whose later memory is to be studied. The items are chosen from two sets, "A" and "B," that have high similarity within sets but low similarity between sets. Following this are two blocks of other items — one of A items, one of B items. Thus one block consists of items whose

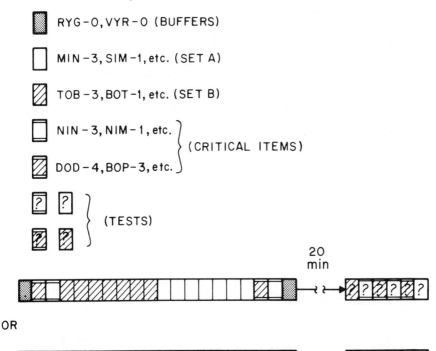

FIGURE 2 Design of experiment demonstrating consolidation in paired-associate learning by a time-dependent, poststimulus interference effect. A key showing item types is given above, the time order of items below. The order of critical items (AB versus BA) at the beginning and end of the series was varied, as was the order of tests. Note that the experimental variable is only the time of occurrence of interfering items relative to critical items (Landauer, 1974).

initial nonsense syllable looks and sounds like that of one critical item. The other block contains nonsense syllables that are as dissimilar as possible from that critical item. Memory for critical items is tested about 20 minutes later. The experimental variation consists in the arrangement of the blocks of items following the critical items. In one experiment we showed that an arrangement in which the more confusable items followed first and then the less confusable produced lower long-term recall than did an arrangement in which the less confusable items followed first and then the more confusable ones. Notice that the critical item was always being recalled in the context of the same set; the only difference was the order in which the items following it appeared.

A comparable effect is not obtained in a forward direction. Consider the critical items at the end of the list, as shown in Figure 2. These critical items

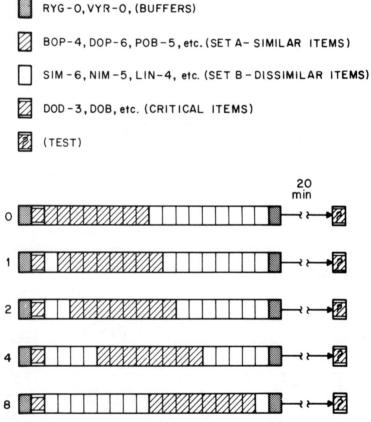

FIGURE 3 Design of experiment showing a temporally graded retrograde effect of interfering items in paired-associate learning. A key showing item types is given above, the time order of items below (Landauer, 1974).

were directly *preceded* by more or less confusable items. No differential effect was obtained. In further experiments we have traced the time after one critical item, or more properly the number of intervening other items, over which the influence occurs. The design for these experiments is shown in Figure 3 and their results in Figure 4. A single critical item was followed by varying numbers of relatively noninterfering items before a block of eight interfering ones was presented. As the number of noninterfering items, and thus the amount of time before disruption increased, the probability of correct cued recall 20 minutes later also increased. The function seems to asymptote at about 6 items, or 60 seconds. One could conclude from this result that the consolidation activity that improves later recall, and is itself interruptable by the presentation of confusable items, is largely completed in less than a minute.

Timing the onset of the effect of alcohol on the nervous system to coincide with this interval would be extremely difficult. It would require, at the very least, some more heroic route of administration than the usual. If the drug took effect before the critical item was presented, one would like to find some way to rule out possible effects on other processes. I doubt this is possible. One might still, however, look for an interaction between effects of delaying interference and those of drug states. If the consolidation initiation phase is shortened under

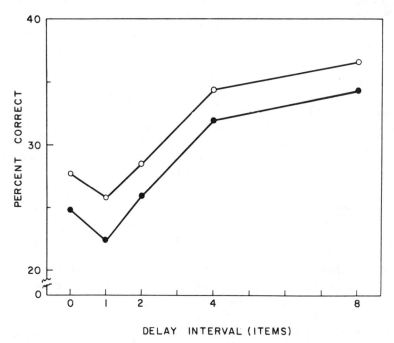

DELAY INTERVAL (ITEMS)

FIGURE 4 Results of experiment described by Figure 3. The two curves are from separate replications. Each point represents data for approximately 175 subjects (Landauer, 1974).

alcohol, for example, a brief interval between critical item and interference might be relatively less disadvantageous in the drugged than in the normal state. But before rushing out to do such an experiment, one should consider the following high stumbling block. The overall level of retention would probably be lower in the drugged state. Consequently, the retrograde interference effect would be measured against different baselines in the two states. It would be very hazardous to interpret absolute differences in percent correct directly because, e.g., there is no justification for believing the difference between 20% and 30% correct to reflect the same change in effectiveness of learning as that between 80% and 90%. However, in the unlikely event that drugged subjects were better with short intervals and worse with long intervals, it would be reasonable to conclude that they have briefer consolidation periods. This kind of scaling problem has been insufficiently recognized in much memory work, especially amnesia research, in which these kinds of interaction experiments are otherwise attractive. Smith (1976) provides a good discussion of the difficulties.

Certain other experiments have suggested that although the first minute after an item is presented is the period during which consolidation can be influenced by interfering verbal material, this does not represent the time during which the actual build-up of the probability of recall takes place.

If the memory for the critical item is measured immediately after the end of the experimental list, instead of after a half-hour, no effect of the variation in order of postpair stimuli is observed. The results of such an experiment are shown in Figure 5. The values at points labeled "mid-point" and "end" are from tests given within the learning list on critical items followed by relatively interfering (I) and noninterfering (N) materials in either IN or NI order. The 20-minute retention data are for similarly treated items that were not tested within the list. (The experiment was slightly different from the paradigm described above. For details see Landauer, 1974.) The results indicate that the effect of retrograde interference is not felt immediately. But after 20 minutes a big effect is obtained. Thus it appears that the variation of when the interfering material is presented which determines how much consolidation will happen must occur within about a minute after the critical item, but that the con-solidation that results does not actually occur until some time later. Unfortu-nately, our experimental attempts to trace in more detail the period during which the effect grows have not been satisfactory. All we know now is what is shown in Figure 5 — that the result grows between 2 minutes and 20.

The distinction between initiating and maturational phases of consolidation may correspond to physiological processes — reverberating conduction activity and biochemical structure manufacture, for example. Evidence suggesting that alcohol-induced memory deficits develop after a half-hour (Goodwin, Othmer, Halikas, & Freemon, 1970) is consistent with a route of alcohol effect that is related to the maturational stage. This hypothesis may be rather directly veri-fiable. If the maturation is relatively continuous over an interval from 2 to at

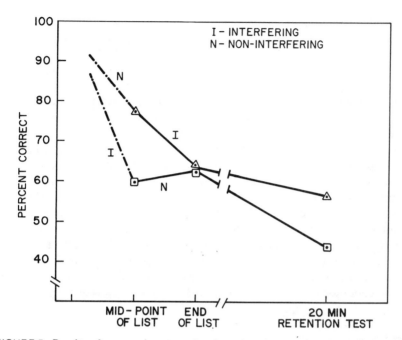

FIGURE 5 Results of an experiment varying the order of poststimulus interference, with independent tests within the list and after 20 minutes. The I and N conditions refer to blocks of relatively easy and dissimilar, or difficult and similar, items. The dashed lines indicate decline in performance from an assumed, but not measured, equal starting point for the two conditions (Landauer, 1974).

least 20 minutes, one could hope to time the onset of the effects of an acute dose of alcohol appropriately to see a retrograde effect. I would be inclined to perform such an experiment by presenting a long list of low-frequency nouns at a very slow rate, say one every 10 seconds. Then at some preselected point, differing for different subjects, administer a dose of alcohol as quickly as possible. One would then compare performance on a free-recall and/or recognition test after one or two days. Items encountered just before alcohol and items received half an hour or more earlier should differ. This would require a list of say 200 to 300 items. If college students were used as subjects, one could expect to observe considerably above-chance performance in the normal state.

Let me discuss now, briefly, the relation of spacing to consolidation, because if I am right, exploring the interaction of drugs with spacing differences would provide another, although probably not as good, way of examining their effects on the initiation phase of consolidation.

In paired associates and a variety of other learning paradigms, two immediately successive presentations of the same item lead to little better long-term retention than does a single presentation; but two well-separated presentations are as much as twice as effective as one presentation. The large number of theories offered to explain this important phenomenon is a tribute to the creativity of modern psychology; a review here is out of the question. One theory, however (Atkinson & Shiffrin, 1968; Landauer, 1969), is that the essential consolidation activity following receipt of an item is all—or—none, or at least rate-limited; so that giving the item again too soon does not help in producing a permanent record. According to most authorities, this theory corresponds to at least as many of the known facts as any other (see, e.g., the review by Hintzman, 1974).

Thus, with some reservation, the spacing effect may be taken as a possible reflection of consolidation initiation. The half value of spacing effects for paired-associate learning is about 30 seconds, giving a second agreeing estimate for the duration of this phase. A drug experiment is fairly obvious. Compare spacing effects for drunk and sober subjects. Of course, the strong caveat discussed above applies; only if intoxicated subjects do better than normals at short spacing intervals and worse at long, would a safe inference be possible. However, the very large effect of spacing suggests that it intimately involves an important mechanism of memory; consequently, exploration of its interaction with alcohol should have a higher expected utility than most such experiments.

Loss Processes

Now, let us continue our survey of methods for tapping processes in Figure 1. Slowly building retroactive interference and autonomous decay, at least if they were treated as a single factor, would be fairly easy to explore. They go on over such a long time period that one could introduce intoxication that was limited to periods in which only these processes are thought to be present.

Retrieval Processes

Retrieval, as a process in itself and as an aspect of input, is another process that deserves more detailed discussion. Some of the experimental literature on alcohol effects suggests that the effects at time of recall are less pronounced than effects at input (e.g., Birnbaum & Parker, this volume). My guess is that alcohol especially dims the ability to register and interpret. There is probably also some amount of dissociation or state dependence. (However, as an aside, some of the experiments that have been taken as demonstration of state dependence are really stronger evidence of an input effect. To my knowledge, wherever an interaction between drug state at time of learning and test has been observed, there has been an even stronger effect of the drug state at time of learning.) But one may still want to ask a further and more detailed question as to whether there is any substantial effect on retrieval, even if it is a smaller effect. What has usually been measured is probability of recall. One might suspect, for various reasons, that the time for retrieval would be a more sensitive and perhaps more important measure. There is precedence for physiological effects on retrieval time in cases where probability correct is not materially affected. Oldfield & Wingfield (1965) studied the function relating word frequency and reaction time to name line drawings of objects for which the words stood. The function was much steeper in brain damaged than in normal patients. Goodwin, Othmer, Halikas and Freemon (1970) observed that subjects under acute alcohol intoxication could remember information from a week before or from their youth as well as sober people. The question is whether reaction-time measurements made under the same conditions may yield different or at least more analytic results.

The nice thing about the word frequency manipulation in particular, as an experimental approach, is that there is good reason to believe that differences in speed as a function of frequency are specifically related to memory search and retrieval processes rather than to input and output processes. The slope of the function reflects retrieval mechanisms, whereas inefficiencies in input and motor response are reflected in its overall height. If one additionally wants to rid this experimental paradigm of special speech-related problems, it can be done in the form of a "lexical decision" task. In this task the subject simply decides whether or not a presented string of letters is an English word. He can do this by saying yes or no or by pulling a lever.

The method has not been applied much yet in alcohol research, but the evidence to date is intriguing. Moskowitz and Roth (1971) found that alcohol increased the effect of word frequency on naming pictures. On the other hand, unpublished data of V. K. Tharp and H. L. Williams, (personal communication, 1976) contain no significant interaction between word frequency and alcohol in naming printed words or repeating spoken words. However, these latter two tasks generally show much smaller frequency effects than does picture naming. One interpretation of this is that in word naming people may often use such response generation processes as grapheme-phoneme correspondence or direct mimicking; and these do not involve access to remembered information about the word as such and thus are not sensitive to its familiarity. Indeed, we have recently found that the same set of words shows a much stronger frequency effect when the task is to decide that a visually presented letter string is a word or that it is not a first name than when the task is to say the word (Landauer, Ross & Didner, 1976). If this analysis is correct, the evidence taken together suggests that alcohol may have a specific effect on memory access after all. More data are needed. The same method could be extended to simple inference-making by asking different kinds of questions. One could ask whether a letter string names something with wings, or someone who lived before 1900, and so forth.

CONCLUDING REMARKS

This brings us to the bottom of Figure 1, and to the end of this review of memory monitoring methods. In closing I would like to make a few remarks on the general issue of research on memory and alcohol. It seems to me that among the human cognitive abilities, that of a rapid, highly cross-referenced, associative memory with large capacity is the most typical and important. It is the cornerstone of them all. The nature of the memory faculty or its degradation by environmental influences, bad habits, or age are consequently issues of almost unexceeded importance.

With special regard to alcohol, there are at least three separable important questions involving memory. First, what acute observable effects on memory are produced by the state of intoxication itself? Are any of these effects larger, deeper, or more dangerous than commonly thought? Second, what are the long-term effects of chronic alcohol use at all levels? Do 20 years of preprandial martinis degrade a person's ability to remember? Third, is there anything about the acute or chronic effects of alcohol on memory that contributes to alcohol dependence? I suppose that the particular interest in the "blackout" phenomenon is partly motivated by such a question, by the hypothesis that amnesia makes it easier to not notice the cues that lead to overdrinking, or not to suffer all its bad consequences. I might suggest that less dramatic effects, as subtle as changes in retrieval time of old information, might conceivably have similar effects. Research with more sensitive methods is needed. Their development could be as worthwhile as anything psychology has ever attempted. That we have sophisticated means for diagnosing the onset of vascular disorders and monitoring them so that we can do research on their causes, but have no equal methods for detecting deterioration of memory is a sad state of affairs. If we could take a view of human memory that would, for the occasion, play down differences between conflicting theories and accentuate the commonalities of known phases and effective factors, we might find our present understanding sufficient to developing a useful set of diagnostic methods.

REFERENCES

Atkinson, R. C., & Shiffrin, R. M. Human memory: A proposed system and its control processes. In K. W. Spence & J. T. Spence (Eds.), *The psychology of learning and motivation,* Vol. 2. New York: Academic Press, 1968.

Baddeley, A. D. *The psychology of memory.* New York: Basic Books, 1976.

Bower, G. H. Stimulus sampling theory of encoding variability. In A. W. Melton & E. Martin (Eds.), *Coding processes in human memory.* Washington, D.C.: V. H. Winston & Sons, 1972.

Crowder, R. G. *Principles of learning and memory.* Hillsdale, N.J.: Lawrence Erlbaum Associates, 1976.

Estes, W. K. Statistical theory of distributional phenomena in learning. *Psychological Review*, 1955, *62*, 360–377.

Geiselman, R. E. Semantic positive forgetting: Another cocktail party problem. *Journal of Verbal Learning and Verbal Behavior*, 1975, *14*, 73–81.

Goodwin, D. W., Othmer, E., Halikas, J. A., & Freemon, F. Loss of short-term memory as a predictor of the alcoholic "blackout." *Nature*, 1970, *227*, 201–201.

Hintzman, D. L. Theoretical implications of the spacing effect. In R. L. Solso (Ed.), *Theories in cognitive psychology: The Loyola symposium.* Potomac, Md.: Lawrence Erlbaum Associates, 1974.

Landauer, T. K. Reinforcement as consolidation. *Psychological Review*, 1969, *76*, 82–96.

Landauer, T. K. Consolidation in human memory: Retrograde amnestic effects of confusable items in paired-associate learning. *Journal of Verbal Learning and Verbal Behavior*, 1974, *13*, 45–53.

Landauer, T. K. Memory without organization: Properties of a model with random storage and undirected retrieval. *Cognitive Psychology;* 1975, *7*, 495–531.

Landauer, T. K., Ross, B. H., & Didner, R. M. On seeing, saying and understanding four-letter words. Paper presented at the meeting of the Psychonomic Society, November 1976.

Milner, B. Amnesia following operation on the temporal lobes. In C. W. M. Whitty & O. L. Zangwill (Eds.), *Amnesia.* London: Butterworth, 1966.

Moskowitz, H., & Roth, S. Effect of alcohol on response latency in object naming. *Quarterly Journal of Studies on Alcohol*, 1971, *32*, 969–975.

Oldfield, R. C., & Wingfield, A. Response latencies in naming objects. *Quarterly Journal of Experimental Psychology*, 1965, *17*, 273–281.

Rothkopf, E. Z. Incidental memory for location of information in text. *Journal of Verbal Learning and Verbal Behavior*, 1971, *10*, 608–613.

Shallice, T., & Warrington, E. K. Independent functioning of verbal memory stores: A neuropsychological study. *Quarterly Journal of Experimental Psychology*, 1970, *22*, 261–273.

Smith, J. E. K. Data transformations in analysis of variance. *Journal of Verbal Learning and Verbal Behavior*, 1976, *15*, 339–346.

Sperling, G. The information available in brief visual presentations. *Psychological Monographs*, 1960, *74*(11, Whole No. 498).

Sperling, G. Successive approximations to a model for short-term memory. *Acta Psychologica*, 1967, *27*, 285–292.

Sternberg, S. High-speed scanning in human memory. *Science*, 1966, *153*, 652–654.

Sternberg, S. Memory scanning: Mental processes revealed by reaction-time experiments. *American Scientist*, 1969, *57*, 421–457. (a)

Sternberg, S. The discovery of processing stages: Extension of Donders' method. *Acta Psychologica*, 1969, *30*, 276–315. (b)

Waugh, N. C., & Norman, D. A. Primary memory. *Psychological Review*, 1965, *72*, 89–104.

Wickelgren, W. A. Sparing of short-term memory in an amnestic patient: Implications for a strength theory of memory. *Neuropsychologia*, 1968, *6*, 235–244.

Wickelgren, W. A. Single-trace fragility theory of memory dynamics. *Memory & Cognition*, 1974, *2*, 775–780.

4

What Is Being Counted None the Less?

Marcia K. Johnson

State University of New York at Stony Brook

Every smallest stroke of virtue or of vice leaves its never so little scar. The drunken Rip Van Winkle, in Jefferson's play, excuses himself for every fresh dereliction by saying, "I won't count this time!" Well! he may not count it, and a kind Heaven may not count it; but it is being counted none the less. Down among his nerve cells and fibres the molecules are counting it, registering and storing it up to be used against him when the next temptation comes. Nothing we ever do is, in strict scientific literalness, wiped out [William James, 1892, p. 150].

Aside from the moral here, at least two important ideas are suggested by this passage. First, that any experience leaves a persisting record, even if its effects are not immediately obvious. Therefore, we ought to be able to detect the effects of our experiences with appropriate measures and paradigms. This idea underlies some of the topics that were considered in detail during the conference. For example, a currently important conceptual and methodological problem is sorting out storage from retrieval deficits in memory (e.g., Birnbaum & Parker, this volume). Similarly, research on state-dependent memory and the role of encoding variability and cue-reinstatement in remembering (e.g., Craik; Goodwin; Keppel & Zubrzycki; Weingartner & Murphy; this volume) suggests that "apparent" forgetting may obscure the essential durability of memory traces.

The second, related, and perhaps corollary idea is that repetitions of similar experiences count or cumulate — again, even though it may not be immediately obvious. There have been a number of especially dramatic illustrations of this point, beginning with Ebbinghaus's (1885) delayed relearning procedure, developed to measure the effects of overlearning. Similarly, Hebb (1961) included a repeated digit sequence in a short-term memory task in order to determine whether transient reverberating traces left any permanent structural trace. Haber and Hershenson (1965) found that repetitions of a word presented at durations at which the word could not be "seen" on the first presentation nevertheless resulted in increases in correct identification over trials. More recently, with a lexical decision task, Forbach, Stanners, and Hochhaus (1974) found that people were faster in deciding a letter string was a word the second time it was presented, even with as much as 10 minutes between repetitions (and decisions about 84 intervening items). Obtaining a "priming" effect over such long intervals suggests that it is not necessarily a temporary phenomenon but may also reflect more permanent changes in memory. It is as if "every smallest stroke . . . leaves its never so little scar."

RECORDING EVENT FREQUENCY

It should not surprise us that one of memory's most remarkable characteristics is its incredible responsiveness to the repetition of events. After all, it is the construct that we make responsible for knowing that something is happening *again*. Without this capacity, it's hard to imagine how perception, thought, and actions could be as orderly as they are. Eddington (1935) suggested that "we should [never] have made progress with the problem of inference from our sensory experience, and theoretical physics would never have originated, if it were not that certain regularities and recurrencies are noticeable in sensory experience [p. 8]." Our perceptual/memory systems have evolved mechanisms for exploiting certain regularities in experience. The nature of these mechanisms is a central, unresolved mystery. But somehow recurrencies are kept track of, and knowledge about the relative frequency of events is the basis for a great deal of our information about the world. Indeed, this is almost certainly one cognitive process underlying learning and memory that we share with most other animals.

Results from many learning situations are consistent with the idea of a mechanism for recording event frequency. For example, pigeons will distribute pecks to two keys in proportion to the number of reinforcements on each (Herrnstein, 1961; Rachlin, 1976). Similarly, children's choices between two alternatives often will match the frequency of occurrence of each (e.g., Messick & Solley, 1957). Adults' predictions about which of two candidates or products will be preferred seems largely determined by which of them has been preferred more frequently in the past (Estes, 1976). Sometimes when two or more responses are possible, one eventually will be made all of the time. Examples would be a rat choosing the arm of a maze that always leads to food rather than the arm that never does, or a pigeon consistently pecking the key that requires fewer pecks per reward, or the child "maximizing" the probability of obtaining prizes. Even in these cases, it seems reasonable to assume that the "sensible" choice reflects stored information about the relative frequency of two or more events.

More direct evidence of the availability of recurrence information comes from tasks in which people are asked to estimate the frequency of events such as words in the English language or to estimate experimentally induced "situational" frequency of items (e.g., Hintzman, 1969; Underwood, Zimmerman, & Freund, 1971). Although the exact values of their judgments may be somewhat in error, the relative judgments are impressively accurate. In addition, judgments about the relative frequency of events seem to be rather insensitive to developmental trends. Very young children show functions relating judged frequency to actual frequency that are very similar to those produced by older children (Hasher, personal communication, 1976). This would be expected assuming that information about the relative frequency of occurrence of events in the environment is among the most fundamental information an organism might have about the environment.

In recent theories of memory, frequency has played a major role in analyses of recognition processes. Many interpretations of recognition assume that it is possible because familiar or old items (targets) have accrued greater frequency than unfamiliar or new items (distractors). According to this view, when the items are studied, situational frequency information is stored each time an item is presented and each time it is rehearsed. This results in a distribution of target items that vary somewhat among themselves in situational frequency value. At the time of the recognition test, the memory representation of each item is checked for situational frequency; since, on the average, targets will have greater frequency values than distractors, this information can be used to discriminate between the two classes of items.

This type of analysis has received considerable experimental support (e.g., Underwood, 1972; Underwood & Freund, 1968; 1970; Underwood et al., 1971; Atkinson & Juola, 1972; Fischler & Juola, 1971). Perhaps because of this, even models that propose that recognition sometimes involves a second process (when the discrimination based on frequency information is difficult and the subject is not sure) usually assume that the primary information used for decisions is related to event frequency (e.g., Atkinson & Juola, 1972; Mandler & Boeck, 1974). That a very fundamental mechanism is involved in recognition is again suggested by the fact that recognition performance of children is very similar to that of adults (see Brown, 1975).

ALCOHOL AND RECURRENCE INFORMATION

In short, processes underlying the monitoring of recurrences, the recording of event frequency, and mechanisms controlling the availability of this information are very likely central memory functions. Therefore, in the context of the conference, it seems worthwhile to consider the possible effects of alcohol on recurrence information. Perhaps recording event frequency is a particularly stable memory function, relatively immune to swings of fate such as species-membership, age, or level of intoxication.[1] Thus, an initial hypothesis might be that tasks depending primarily on event frequency information should be little disrupted by moderate doses of alcohol to nonalcoholic subjects, compared to tasks (e.g., free recall, problem solving) requiring other processes. Although this prediction could be based on a model of cognitive functioning involving a hierarchy of processes ranging from the "automatic" to the "strategic,"[2] this hypothesis might also be derived from the faith that a kind Heaven would see to it that something so useful to survival as recording recurrence information would be the last to go.

This general notion receives some encouragement from the suggestion by Parker, Alkana, Birnbaum, Hartley, and Noble (1974) that perhaps "the more demanding the task the greater the impairment from alcohol [p. 826]." Presumably, demanding tasks are those that involve finding or generating associations, interrelationships, or structures so that the recall of one event leads to the recall of another, and undemanding tasks are those that capitilize on the propensity of our molecules for recording experienced events.

Although a fairly wide range of tasks have been used in investigations of the effects of alcohol on memory (Ryback, 1971), most of them require reproduction of the target material. There do not seem to be any studies requiring subjects to make either absolute or relative judgments about the frequency of events. It would be interesting to have the results of experiments specifically directed at the question of whether recurrences cumulate as effectively under alcohol conditions as they normally do. Similar relative judgments among items

---

[1] Of course, *how* events are defined (i.e., what constitutes an "event") may vary widely across species, age groups, or levels of intoxication. The present discussion by-passes this difficult, but interesting, problem.

[2] For example, Brown (1975) makes a distinction between "memory facilitated by strategic intervention" and memory that is an "involuntary product of our continuous interactions with a relatively meaningful environment [p. 113]." Craik and Lockhart (1972) note that "after the stimulus has been recognized, it may undergo further processing by enrichment or elaboration." In the levels of processing framework proposed by Craik and Lockhart, "trace persistence is a function of depth of analysis, with deeper levels of analysis associated with more elaborate, longer lasting, and stronger traces [p. 675]." In contrast, here it is assumed that all memory traces are durable, but under some conditions, it may be more difficult to detect some of them than others. For example, organizational and elaborative processes produce traces or sets of interrelated traces that perhaps make it easier for subjects to recall information as compared to the traces produced by processes involved in recording recurrences. However, this does not mean that more embellished traces are necessarily longer lasting than less embellished traces. Regardless of the details of the particular models or classification schemes, discussions such as Brown's and Craik and Lockhart's emphasize the importance of acknowledging the variety of mental activities that may occur when a stimulus is presented and the importance of clarifying *which* processes are critical to a given type of performance and which are subject to disruption from various experimental treatments.

of differing frequencies under alcohol and control conditions would indicate a continued functioning of processes involved in recording recurrences. Less directly, it might also be possible to determine whether subjects profit as much under alcohol conditions from repeating "right" items in a verbal discrimination learning task (e.g., Underwood, Jesse, & Ekstrand, 1964).

Although frequency judgments are not available, there have been several alcohol studies employing recognition paradigms. One interesting finding that at first fits nicely into the "kind Heaven" hypothesis is that measures of memory based on recognition seem to be less susceptible to state-dependent effects than do measures of memory based on recall (Goodwin, Powell, Bremer, Hoine, & Stern, 1969; Osborn, cited in Overton, 1972; Wickelgren, 1975; see also Eich, this volume). You may not be able to recall all of the people at that cocktail party last night, but you have a fair chance of recognizing them the next day.

Although recognition may not show state-dependent effects, there does seem to be an overall decrement in recognition as alcohol dose is increased (Goodwin et al., 1969; Ryback, Weinert, & Fozard, 1970; Wickelgren, 1975; Birnbaum & Parker, this volume). However, before we conclude that alcohol does disrupt the recording of recurrence information we should consider some of the other possible sources of this decrement in recognition.

One possibility is that alcohol makes it less likely that the interpretation or representation activated during the test is the same as that activated during the study trial (e.g., Light & Carter-Sobell, 1970; Tulving & Thomson, 1973; Hasher & Johnson, 1975; Hashtroudi & Johnson, 1976). If the appropriate trace is not contacted, the appropriate recurrence information will not be available. Some evidence regarding this notion may be obtained from studies in which subjects are asked to generate associates to stimuli and are later asked again to generate the same associates (Goodwin et al., 1969; Weingartner & Faillace, 1971). Although Weingartner and Faillace did not find any impairment in retention of previously given associates from administering alcohol to nonalcoholic subjects, Goodwin et al. did. Insofar as associates give some clue about the stability of encoding of an item, this paradigm is quite interesting. For now, evidence for less stability in the *basic* encoding of stimuli under alcohol does not seem overwhelming; this is consistent with the failure to find marked state-dependent effects with recognition. If the encoding of an item is relatively stable from alcohol to nonalcohol state and vice versa, then it seems likely that it would be relatively stable across two presentations under alcohol.

More central to the present discussion is the possibility that alcohol reduces attention to the stimuli and thus not as many are experienced as in the control condition. Frequency increments cannot accrue to representations that are not activated. That this might not be the entire source of the poorer performance, however, is suggested by the fact that Wickelgren (1975) found a small but significant decrement in recognition with a continuous procedure that required subjects to respond to every item.

Another possibility is that sober subjects may rehearse more during acquisition and thus generate more frequency increments.[3] Covert rehearsal is something that is generally difficult to equate across conditions, but it is critical where tests of frequency effects in recognition are concerned (Raye, 1976). Using incidental orienting tasks during acquisition (e.g., Craik, this volume) might be one technique to guarantee processing of every input, and it might also serve to equate uncontrolled rehearsals in alcohol and control subjects.

In speculating about other factors that might contribute to a recognition decrement, it is worth considering the source of errors — especially false positives — in recognition. There is some evidence that false positives are a consequence of the implicit activation of distractors during acquisition (Underwood, 1965; Kimble, 1968). That is, during study, not only are representations of the presented items activated, but so are ideas that may be associated with the targets. Thoughts other than those directly representing the stimuli are taking place. And, although these thoughts may be conscious, they are not necessarily so. If some of these previously activated associations are among the distractors they may seem familiar, and the subject will make false positive responses. Suppose alcohol increases the number of different implicit responses (i.e., produces less focused thinking) during acquisition. This would increase the difficulty of subsequently rejecting any given set of distractors. Or suppose alcohol produces a tendency during acquisition to give relatively more attention to internally generated events and relatively less to externally generated events. Distractors should then have relatively more frequency increments and targets relatively less, producing not only increased false positives but also decreased hits.

The above discussion has included three main points:

1. We do not have much information about whether recurrences are recorded as well under alcohol as control conditions. If they are not, this would indicate that a very central memory function is disrupted by alcohol. Furthermore, such a disruption could certainly account for a recognition decrement if recognition is based primarily on frequency information. Available data does not allow us to confidently reject the hypothesis that alcohol does not affect recording event frequency.

2. Even if alcohol does not affect the reliability or sensitivity with which recurrence information is recorded, alcohol and control conditions could differ in the number of functional occurrences of target items. That is, thinking again about (or internally generating) recent events is the sort of "self-initiated set" (Parsons & Prigatano, this volume) like semantic elaboration or organization,

---

[3] As previously stated, the assumption of frequency models of recognition is that covert activations of ideas result in frequency increments that may be included in estimates of perceptual event frequency. Some evidence regarding this assumption will be presented later.

which seems most easily disrupted by alcohol. (In this regard, Goodwin, this volume, reported a procedure in which reminding subjects about a recent event during a blackout considerably reduced the usual forgetting obtained.) In fact, organizing information probably depends on a set to and the ability to covertly generate previously presented items.

3. Alcohol may affect the number (or range) of occurrences of internally generated items that are *not* part of the target set. Thus one important effect of alcohol may be that it changes what is available to be counted by a recurrence mechanism.

THE PROBLEM OF REALITY-MONITORING

However, as soon as we assume that there are two types of events taking place at acquisition — the activation or establishment of memory traces that more or less directly represent the external stimuli and those that represent other ideas — a critical problem is highlighted. How do we discriminate between these two types of representations? To the extent that this discrimination occurs, a thought might not provoke a false positive during a recognition test no matter how many frequency increments it had accrued. Conversely, any manipulation that makes this discrimination more difficult should increase recognition errors. Thus another possibility (which does not necessarily exclude any of those discussed previously) is that alcohol somehow decreases a person's ability to discriminate the memories generated by perceptual experience from those generated by other processes. The type and frequency of externally and internally generated representations might be similar under alcohol and control conditions, but telling the difference between them later ("reality-monitoring") may be more difficult in the former case.[4] It seems plausible that drinking alcohol might impair a person's ability to distinguish fact from fantasy. (An understandable motivation for social drinking!) Recognition tests are situations in which fairly stringent criteria for distinguishing memories for external and internal events are appropriate, because internally generated items that were not on the target list represent potential errors. If alcohol lowers these criteria, increases in false positives would be expected.

Whether only false positives should increase, or whether hits might be affected also, depends on how the memory representations of external and internal events differ. If memories for thoughts and memories for perceptual "facts"

---

[4] The problem of distinguishing fact from fantasy has received special attention in the context of certain clinical problems, such as schizophrenia, and the process by which this is accomplished is sometimes called "reality testing" (e.g., Cameron, 1963). Reality-monitoring is intended to be a more neutral term with respect to the underlying mechanisms for the same general capacity. In addition, "monitoring" also has the connotation (appropriate here) of making judgments about *past* events represented in memory (Hart, 1967).

differ in that thoughts are on the average simply weaker versions of facts, then perhaps lowered criteria should increase both false positives and hits. On the other hand, if they differ more on qualitative dimensions, a shift in criteria would not necessarily have parallel effects on hits and false positives. Including a wider range of types of memory representations in the "acceptable category" might produce an increase in false positives while leaving hits relatively unchanged. Unfortunately, hits and false positives are often not reported separately. In general, this would be interesting information to preserve in reporting recognition results since it might provide some clues about the nature of the effects of specific experimental manipulations.

In discussing results of studies of people with severe amnesia, Warrington and Weiskrantz (1970, 1971) suggested these subjects may "fail to categorise separately the 'new' and the 'old', or ... there is a tendency for over-generalisation among the alternative items in store [1971, p. 67]." They used a technique in which visually degraded versions of word stimuli were used as cues for recall. As compared to normal subjects, the amnesic subjects did comparatively worse in a standard yes/no recognition task than in the cued procedure. Warrington and Weiskrantz proposed that the cuing technique helped eliminate interference from false positives that occurs in the recognition situation. Their notion of overgeneralization among alternative stored items is similar to the present idea regarding potential effects of moderate doses of alcohol on reality-monitoring, if it is assumed that some of the overgeneralization is between stored representations of external events and stored representations of internal events.

As has been argued elsewhere (Johnson, 1975; Johnson, Taylor, & Raye, 1977), knowledge about the similarities and differences in memories established by perceptual experience and those established primarily via other processes is critical to an adequate theory of memory. Under ordinary circumstances, most of us are reasonably good at sorting out fact and fantasy. For example, subjects rarely intrude their elaborators and mnemonic devices during recall tasks. On the other hand, there certainly are circumstances in which the two are confused and thus the processes that operate to distinguish between memories for fact and for fantasy and the conditions under which they break down are potentially quite interesting.

Carol Raye and I, and some of the students working with us,[5] have been trying to develop a procedure to study confusion between occurrence information for perceptually and internally derived events. We started with the assumption that in order to conclude that the memory representation of an imagination (or internally generated information) has been confused with the memory representation of a perception, both the imagination and the perception must have occurred prior to the test. Our basic paradigm involved manipulating the number

[5] I would especially like to acknowledge the valuable help of Thomas H. Taylor and Alvin Y. Wang with some of the studies mentioned here.

of times various items were presented and manipulating the number of times subjects produced these items (either overtly or covertly) during the first phase of the experiment. After this, subjects were asked to estimate either the number of times each item had been presented or the number of times they had generated each item.

For example, in one experiment, 36 items were formed using the name of 36 Battig and Montague (1969) categories as cues and one high frequency instance of each category as to-be-remembered items (Johnson et al., 1977). On a study trial, 18 cue—item pairs were presented; on any given test trial 18 cues were presented and the subjects wrote down the appropriate item in the blank beside each cue. Study and test trials alternated, and individual items were studied a total of either 2, 5, or 8 times and were tested a total of either 2, 5, or 8 times. The sequence of studying and testing items was random, except, of course, for the restriction that no item was tested before it had been studied. Following this phase of the experiment, subjects were presented with each item individually, and half were asked to estimate how many times each word had been presented and half were asked to estimate how many times they generated each word.

The data for those subjects asked to judge the number of presentations are shown in Figure 1. As can be seen, the mean judged frequency of occurrence of

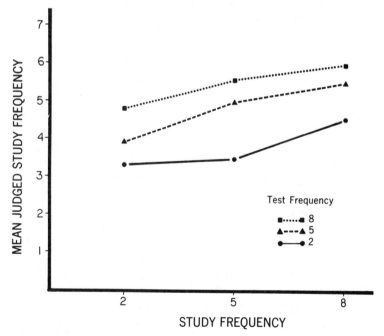

FIGURE 1 Judged study frequency as a function of manipulated study frequency. Each line represents a different test frequency. (From Johnson, M. K., Taylor, T. H., & Raye, C. L., *Memory & Cognition*, 1977, 5, 116–122. Reprinted by permission.)

items increased as the actual frequency of occurrence increased. This replicates previous findings and indicates that subjects are sensitive to the relative frequency of external events in the context of the present procedure. The separation between the lines in Figure 1 indicates that the number of times subjects produced the items resulted in increases in the apparent frequency of occurrence of the items. We call this increase in apparent frequency of external events as a consequence of internally generated events the IFE effect.

Although at first it may be tempting to suppose that the IFE effect is a consequence of writing the items down (and thus as the subject reads his own production another "external" event takes place), we have also found this basic effect under a number of conditions where subjects do not overtly produce the items. For example, we have had subjects covertly produce the words and simply indicate with a check whether or not they could remember them, or subjects have been asked to imagine a representation of the items and rate the vividness of their images. Both of these conditions also produce an increase in apparent frequency as internally generated occurrences increase (Johnson et al., 1977). Similarly, the effect is obtained with picture stimuli and test trials during which the subject attempts to image the pictures (Johnson & Raye, 1976). Thus the assumption in the previous discussion of recognition that implicit activations result in frequency increments that may be included in estimates of external event frequency is confirmed by these data.

The mean scores of those subjects asked to estimate the number of times they produced each item are shown in Figure 2. Estimates of generation frequency increased with actual increases in test frequency. This provides evidence that subjects are sensitive to the relative frequency of internally generated events. In addition, increases in the number of presentations contributed to the apparent frequency of productions. We call this increase in the apparent frequency of internally generated events as a consequence of externally generated events the IFI effect.

Overall, these findings indicate that we have a remarkably sensitive cumulative record not only of external events but of internal events as well. In addition, our data provide direct evidence for confusion between externally and internally generated events in that each increased the apparent frequency of the other. Given the previous discussion and the above data, several questions are suggested.

First, is frequency information for external and internal events disrupted by alcohol, and, if so, are they disrupted equally? Is alcohol more or less likely to affect the way in which similar externally generated experiences cumulate than the way in which similar internally generated experiences cumulate? From this information we might be able, for example, to develop some predictions about whether intoxicated people are more likely to remember acts they initiate or acts initiated by others, or whether they are more likely to recognize repetitions in their own thoughts and behavior or repetitions in the behavior of others.

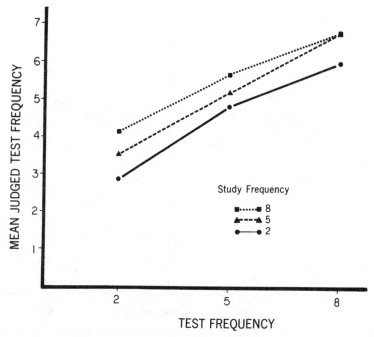

FIGURE 2 Judged test frequency as a function of manipulated test frequency. Each line represents a different study frequency. (From Johnson, M. K., Taylor, T. H., & Raye, C. L., *Memory & Cognition,* 1977, 5, 116–122. Reprinted by permission.)

Secondly, is reality-monitoring affected by alcohol? In general, the criteria for distinguishing among internally and externally generated events may vary from situation to situation. For example, depending on the material or task, subjects may adopt more stringent or more lenient criteria for including a representation in their "frequency count." Alcohol may be a treatment that affects the criteria for distinguishing memories for thoughts from those for perceptions. If so, increasing doses of alcohol should increase the extent to which internally generated productions add to the apparent frequency of items in our paradigm (see Figure 3).

Third, are some people more susceptible than others to a breakdown of reality-monitoring? It seems reasonable to suppose that, under usual conditions, the ability to distinguish internally generated events from externally generated events differs from individual to individual. And perhaps some people are less likely than others to have this capacity disrupted by alcohol. Consistent with this idea is Ryback et al.'s (1970) noting the large individual differences in disruption of recognition performance from alcohol in their study. A finding that would be particularly interesting in light of the present discussion would be that people showing relatively small IFE effects in our paradigm under sober

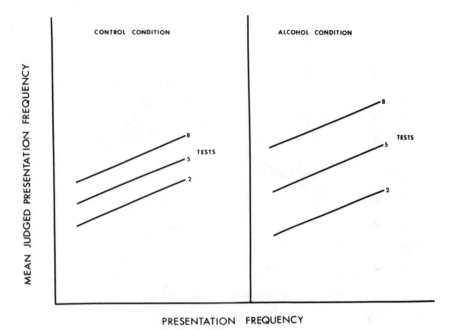

FIGURE 3 Hypothetical data showing a greater increase in the apparent frequency of external events as a consequence of internally generated events (IFE effect) in alcohol than in control conditions.

conditions might also show less effect of alcohol on recognition performance. (On the general importance of individual differences in alcohol research, see also Bahrick, this volume; Jones & Jones, this volume.)

In summary, recording recurrences of events is a fundamental function of memory. Studies of the effects of alcohol on judgments of both external and internal event frequency might augment available information about the types of processes that are susceptible to alcohol disruption. In addition, the paradigm we have been using perhaps could be adapted to alcohol studies to provide evidence about whether alcohol increases confusion between externally and internally generated events. Such a finding might also have implications for analyses of the effects of alcohol on recognition.

A more complete understanding of the source of recognition decrements might also be useful in understanding recall data. In many analyses of recall, recognition tacitly or explicitly plays a role. For example, generate-and-recognize models of recall postulate two distinct phases in the recall process: (1) retrieval of instances that are then (2) evaluated via a recognition process (e.g., Martin, 1975). Thus in recall, the problem of how a person "knows" a retrieved item is a correct item is sometimes relegated to the recognition process. Alcohol might affect not only the processes responsible for retrieving items but might also increase confusion among retrieved items that were and were not on the target list. This should result in a greater number of intrusions in recall (there is some hint of this in Kalin, 1964).

Other consequences of increased confusion between externally and internally generated events from drinking alcohol might be an increase in reports of previous thoughts as having been articulated or acted upon, a tendency to attribute to others things they did not say, and perhaps a breakdown in coordinated conversations because a person does not accurately monitor expressed vs. unexpressed thoughts during the conversation. Parker et al. (1974) mentioned a study by R. C. Smith in which "subjects showed decreased acknowledgment to another's response in conversations [p. 827]." While this certainly could reflect a failure to store or retrieve the other person's comments, or simply bad manners, it would also be consistent with some of the above speculations.

REFERENCES

Atkinson, R. C., & Juola, J. F. Search and decision processes in recognition memory, Technical Report No. 194, Psychology and Education series. Institute for Mathematical Studies in the Social Sciences, Stanford University, 1972.

Battig, W. F., & Montague, W. E. Category norms for verbal items in 56 categories: A replication and extension of the Connecticut category norms. *Journal of Experimental Psychology Monograph*, 1969, *80*, (3, Part 2).

Brown, A. L. The development of memory: Knowing, knowing about knowing, and knowing how to know. In H. W. Reese (Ed.), *Advances in child development and behavior*. (Vol. 10). New York: Academic Press, 1975.

Cameron, N. A. *Personality development and psychopathology: A dynamic approach.* Boston: Houghton-Mifflin, 1963.

Craik, F. I. M., & Lockhart, R. S. Levels of processing: A framework for memory research. *Journal of Verbal Learning and Verbal Behavior*, 1972, *11*, 671–684.

Ebbinghaus, H. *Über das gedachtnis.* Leipzig: Duncker & Humblot, 1885. (Reissued by Dover Publications, 1964.)

Eddington, A. *New pathways in science.* Cambridge, England: University Press, 1935.

Estes, W. K. The cognitive side of probability learning. *Psychological Review*, 1976, *83*, 37–64.

Fischler, I., & Juola, J. F. Effects of repeated tests on recognition time for information in long-term memory. *Journal of Experimental Psychology*, 1971, *91*, 54–58.

Forbach, G. B., Stanners, R. F., & Hochhaus, L. Repetition and practice effects in a lexical decision task. *Memory & Cognition*, 1974, *2*, 337–339.

Goodwin, D. W., Powell, B., Bremer, D., Hoine, H., & Stern, J. Alcohol and recall: State-dependent effects in man. *Science*, 1969, *163*, 1358–1360.

Haber, R. N., & Hershenson, M. Effects of repeated brief exposures on the growth of a percept. *Journal of Experimental Psychology*, 1965, *69*, 40–46.

Hart, J. T. Memory and the memory-monitoring process. *Journal of Verbal Learning and Verbal Behavior*, 1967, *6*, 685–691.

Hasher, L., & Johnson, M. K. Interpretive factors in forgetting. *Journal of Experimental Psychology: Human Learning and Memory*, 1975, *1*, 567–575.

Hashtroudi, S., & Johnson, M. K. Transfer and forgetting: Interpretive shifts and stimulus reinstatement. *Journal of Experimental Psychology: Human Learning and Memory*, 1976, *2*, 262–272.

Hebb, D. O. Distinctive features of learning in the higher animal. In J. F. Delafresnaye (Ed.), *Brain mechanisms and learning*. London: Oxford University Press, 1961.

Herrnstein, R. J. Relative and absolute strength of response as a function of frequency of reinforcement. *Journal of the Experimental Analysis of Behavior*, 1961, *4*, 267–272.

Hintzman, D. L. Apparent frequency as a function of frequency and the spacing of repetitions. *Journal of Experimental Psychology*, 1969, *80*, 139–145.

James, W. *Psychology: Briefer course*. New York: Henry Holt and Company, 1892.

Johnson, M. K. Constructive aspects of memory: Historical antecedents. Paper presented at the annual meeting of the American Psychological Association, Chicago, September 1975.

Johnson, M. K., & Raye, C. L. Fact and fantasy: Confusion between perceptual experiences and imaginations. Annual meeting of the Psychonomic Society, St. Louis, November 1976.

Johnson, M. K., Taylor, T. H., & Raye, C. L. Fact and fantasy: The effects of internally generated events on the apparent frequency of externally generated events. *Memory and Cognition*, 1977, *5*, 116–122.

Kalin, R. Effects of alcohol on memory. *Journal of Abnormal and Social Psychology*, 1964, *69*, 635–641.

Kimble, G. A. Mediating associations. *Journal of Experimental Psychology*, 1968, *76*, 263–266.

Light, L. L., & Carter-Sobell, L. Effects of changed semantic context on recognition memory. *Journal of Verbal Learning and Verbal Behavior*, 1970, *9*, 1–11.

Mandler, G., & Boeck, W. J. Retrieval processes in recognition. *Memory & Cognition*, 1974, *2*, 613–615.

Martin, E. Generation–recognition theory and the encoding specificity principle. *Psychological Review*, 1975, *82*, 150–153.

Messick, S. J., & Solley, C. M. Probability learning in children: Some exploratory studies. *Journal of Genetic Psychology*, 1957, *90*, 23–32.

Overton, D. A. State-dependent learning produced by alcohol and its relevance to alcoholism. In B. Kissin & H. Begleiter (Eds.), *The biology of alcoholism: Physiology and Behavior* (Vol. 2). New York: Plenum Press, 1972.

Parker, E. S., Alkana, R. L., Birnbaum, I. M., Hartley, J. T., & Noble, E. P. Alcohol and the disruption of cognitive processes. *Archives of General Psychiatry*, 1974, *31*, 824–828.

Rachlin, H. C. *Behavior and learning*. San Francisco: W. H. Freeman and Company, 1976.

Raye, C. L. Recognition: Frequency or organization? *American Journal of Psychology*, 1976, *89*, 645–658.

Ryback, R. S. The continuum and specificity of the effects of alcohol on memory. A review. *Quarterly Journal of Studies on Alcohol*, 1971, *32*, 995–1016.

Ryback, R. S., Weinert, J., & Fozard, J. L. Disruption of short-term memory in man following consumption of ethanol. *Psychonomic Science*, 1970, *20*, 353–354.

Tulving, E., & Thomson, D. M. Encoding specificity and retrieval processes in episodic memory. *Psychological Review*, 1973, *80*, 352–373.

Underwood, B. J. False recognition produced by implicit verbal responses. *Journal of Experimental Psychology*, 1965, *70*, 122–129.

Underwood, B. J. Word recognition memory and frequency information. *Journal of Experimental Psychology*, 1972, *94*, 276–283.

Underwood, B. J., & Freund, J. S. Errors in recognition learning and retention. *Journal of Experimental Psychology*, 1968, *78*, 55–63.

Underwood, B. J., & Freund, J. S. Testing effects in the recognition of words. *Journal of Verbal Learning and Verbal Behavior,* 1970, *9,* 117–125.

Underwood, B. J., Jesse, F., & Ekstrand, B. R. Knowledge of rights and wrongs in verbal-discrimination learning. *Journal of Verbal Learning and Verbal Behavior,* 1964, *3,* 183–186.

Underwood, B. J., Zimmerman, J., & Freund, J. S. Retention of frequency information with observations on recognition and recall. *Journal of Experimental Psychology,* 1971, *87,* 149–162.

Warrington, E. K., & Weiskrantz, L. Amnesic syndrome: Consolidation or retrieval? *Nature,* 1970, *228,* 628–630.

Warrington, E. K., & Weiskrantz, L. Organisational aspects of memory in amnesic patients. *Neuropsychologia,* 1971, *9,* 67–73.

Weingartner, H., & Faillace, L. A. Alcohol state-dependent learning in man. *Journal of Nervous and Mental Disease,* 1971, *153,* 395–406.

Wickelgren, W. A. Alcoholic intoxication and memory storage dynamics. *Memory & Cognition,* 1975, *3,* 385–389.

5

Reliability of Measurement in Investigations of Learning and Memory

Harry P. Bahrick

Ohio Wesleyan University

Dependability of observation has been a key concern of investigators since the beginning of scientific inquiry. Variability of the dependent variable unrelated to the manipulated variables must be specified and limited. Such residual "noise effects" reflect imperfections of control that define and limit progress toward the scientific goal of establishing invariant relations.

Whether a given variable contributes toward signal or noise depends, of course, upon the objectives and design of the research. Fluctuations due to apparatus variability, procedural change, experimenter behavior, and momentary states of the subject are usually among the sources of unreliability, unless these variables themselves become the object of inquiry and are manipulated in an investigation designed to test their influence. Variations due to individual differences among subjects affect the results of virtually all psychological research, but they are components of the error term only in those investigations that seek to establish principles of behavior that apply to the population. In contrast, they become the focus of interest in most research concerned with the development of psychological tests. In such research, investigators seek to maximize variation associated with individual differences while attempting to minimize variation of performance of the individual subjects.

Applied psychologists, particularly those working in the field of tests and measurements, not only specify reliability of their measures; they also set explicit, high standards in regard to tolerable levels of unreliability. They routinely lengthen or modify tests until the required reliability is achieved. In contrast, experimental psychologists have paid scant attention to this fundamental problem. Although the statistical significance of treatment effects is assured by tests of statistical inference, acceptable standards of reliability for individual indicants are rarely discussed, and little or no research is directed at the objective of improving the reliability of individual techniques or measures. The correlational approach common in research concerned with individual differences, but unpopular in most areas of experimental psychology, helps to differentiate between statistical and practical significance. Variables are of practical significance if they account for a substantial portion of variance on dependent measures, not if they account for a variance significantly larger than error variance. This type of assessment of variables is lacking in most areas of experimental psychology, and methods of measurement continue to be employed with little regard to their susceptibility to noise effects, i.e., to the magnitude of error terms associated with their use.

The main purpose of this paper is to call attention to this problem by demonstrating in two areas of learning and memory research that minor modifications of procedure may result in marked change in the error variance associated with the dependent measures. Clearly such variations of reliability have a direct bearing upon the power and validity of empirical work, and some of the implications in regard to the analysis of cognitive processes will be discussed.

THE RELIABILITY OF RECOGNITION TESTS

The first group of dependent measures to be examined involves tests of recognition memory. Four commonly used techniques of testing recognition of a previously exposed word list were compared. The four techniques differ in regard to two characteristics defining the test situation. One characteristic involves simultaneous vs. successive presentation of the test material; the other involves specification vs. nonspecification of the number of target items the subject must select. The four possible combinations of these dichotomies yield a 2 X 2 design in which each combination corresponds to a commonly used version of recognition test procedure: simultaneous presentation with specified number of target items (SIM–SPEC); simultaneous presentation with unspecified number of target items (SIM–UN); successive presentation with specified number of target items (SUC–SPEC); and successive presentation with unspecified number of target items (SUC–UN).

The material used consisted of 240 two-syllable nouns selected randomly from every fifth page of the Thorndike–Lorge (1944) list. Sixty of the words were randomly selected as the learning material; the remaining 180 words were used as distractors on the recognition tests. The subjects were 96 male and female Ohio Wesleyan University undergraduates who were trained individually and were instructed to learn the words on the list without regard to their sequence. No information was given about the length of the list. The list was exposed on a memory drum at a rate of 1 word per second. Three exposure trials were given, with an intertrial interval of 10 seconds, and a different random sequence of the words was used for each trial. Immediately following the last trial subjects were instructed to count backward from 60 by 3's; this filler task was used to control recency effects. Twenty-four subjects were assigned by systematic alternation to each of the four testing conditions. The tests were administered immediately after subjects completed the filler task.

In the SIM–SPEC condition the subjects were shown a list of 120 words that included the 60 target words and 60 foils in random order. They were instructed to identify the 60 previously exposed words, to guess if necessary, but to make 60 responses. A 10-minute time limit was imposed, with a warning given at the end of 8 minutes if subjects had not completed the test. In the SIM–UN condition the same material and procedure was used as in the SIM–SPEC condition, with the exception that no mention was made of the number of required responses, and no guessing instructions were given. Subjects were told to identify the words they recognized from the previously exposed list. In the SUC–UN condition the same 120 words were presented individually in random order at a 5-second rate, and subjects were instructed to classify each word as old or new, depending upon whether or not they recognized the word as a member of the previously exposed list. No instructions were added in regard to guessing. In the SUC–SPEC condition the test consisted of 60 multiple-choice items presented individually in random sequence. Each multiple-choice item consisted of a target word and three foils, and subjects were instructed to identify the target word and to guess if necessary. Ten seconds were allowed for each response. Four alternatives rather than two alternatives were used in each multiple-choice item, because preliminary data indicated that recognition performance with a two-alternative version was higher than performance with the other testing conditions and that ceiling effects would limit the validity of variance comparisons.

Table 1 shows the mean number of correct responses in each of the four testing conditions and the variance among the 24 subjects tested in each condition. These values are also shown after each subject's score was corrected

TABLE 1
Performance on Recognition Tests Under Four Testing Conditions

Test condition	Mean number correct		Variance	
	Uncorrected	Corrected	Uncorrected	Corrected
SIM–SPEC	51.2	42.6	12.5	33.1
SIM–UN	47.0	43.3	88.5	125.3
SUC–SPEC	50.0	47.0	40.7	48.0
SUC–UN	46.7	43.2	66.1	68.0

for guessing. The correction was made by subtracting the number of false positive responses from the number of correct positive responses (right − wrong) for all subjects except those who served in the SUC–SPEC condition.[1] The correction formula used for the SUC–SPEC condition was right − $\frac{1}{3}$ wrong, since the number of foils was three times as large as the number of target items.

Inspection of the uncorrected values in Table 1 shows that mean performance is fairly comparable, but variances differ by a ratio of more than 7:1. The modification of Bartlett's test described by Dixon and Massey (1969, p. 309) yields F (3,120) = 8.89 ($p < .001$). The same test applied to the data after the guessing corrections are made yields F (3,120) = 3.71 ($p < .02$). An F_{max} test yields F (4,23) = 7.08 ($p < .001$) and F (4,23) = 3.78 ($p < .02$) for the uncorrected and for the corrected data respectively.

Inspection of Table 1 shows that the variance differences are primarily a function of whether the number of responses to be made is specified or unspecified, and not whether the items are presented simultaneously or successively.

The variance reduction achieved by specifying the number of responses can be understood by regarding the total number of correct positive responses as a joint function of the number of items retained and the number of items correctly guessed. If a fixed number of responses is required, guessing is limited to the difference between the specified number of responses and the number of items the subject has retained. A subject who is required to make 60 responses and who has accurate retention of 58 items will guess at 2 items, regardless of what his general inclinations about guessing might be; and a subject who has accurate retention of 40 items will guess at 20 items. Thus the amount of guessing is limited, and a high negative correlation is introduced between the amount of retention and the amount of guessing. In contrast, if the number of responses is left unspecified, no limit is imposed on guessing; the correlation between amount of retention and amount of guessing is undetermined; and the amount of guessing is a function of unknown subject characteristics.

The addition of a random guessing component to a set of scores increases variance among the scores, but the addition of a negatively correlated guessing component reduces variance, since small amounts are added to large scores, and large amounts to small scores. The lower variance associated with conditions of specified number of responses can be understood on this basis. Although all forms of guessing include random success components, in the specified response

---

[1] It can be argued that the correction for the simultaneous exposure conditions should be smaller, because subjects will begin to guess only after they identified the target items of which they are certain. After target items have been eliminated in this way, the remaining pool of items contains more foils than target items, and therefore guessing produces fewer chance successes. Guessing corrections based upon such rationale are smaller than those used in Table 1. As a result the significance of variance differences among the four conditions increases beyond the level reported in the text.

conditions, guessing adds a comparatively smaller random component and a large negatively correlated component. The net effect is a reduction of variance among subjects.

The correction for guessing reduces scores by subtracting a statistical estimate based upon the number of wrong responses. As a result of this correction the variance of the residual scores will increase if the amount of guessing was negatively correlated with the amount of knowledge. This increase occurs, because high scores are reduced by small amounts and low scores by large amounts. It can be seen that the guessing correction caused a relatively greater increase of variance for the specified response conditions, and this reflects the large negative correlation between the amount of retention and the amount of guessing characteristic of these conditions. Despite the effect of this correction the variance among corrected scores remains significantly smaller for the SIM—SPEC condition. This will be true so long as the knowledge component is large in comparison to the guessing component, so that the average amount of guessing is smaller than under the unspecified response conditions. Thus the advantage of specifying the number of responses is that it limits the amount of guessing to the difference between the number of remembered items and the number of specified responses. If this difference is sufficiently small, the average amount of guessing will be smaller than under conditions where no limit is imposed, and reductions of variance will be effected as in the present case.

Specification of the number of responses is more effective in reducing variance when the items are presented simultaneously than when they are presented successively. This interaction may reflect less variability of guessing in the successive presentation conditions. The reduced effect of guessing in the SUC—SPEC condition is, of course, a function of the larger number of foils, but the enhancement of the knowledge component that necessitated the use of a larger number of foils for this condition reflects the advantage to the subject of limiting the required discrimination on the recognition test. An analogy can be made with the paired-comparison procedure of obtaining a rank order. This procedure generally improves reliability of the obtained order, because it limits all comparisons to two items. In the SUC—SPEC condition the knowledge component can be used more effectively, because the required discriminations are similarly limited. In the SUC—UN condition this advantage is lost, as can be seen from the corrected mean; however, variance is lower than in the SIM—UN condition, perhaps because the SUC—UN test version forces the subject to attend to each item for an equal amount of time under comparable conditions.

The data in Table 1 show that guessing corrections can increase the within-group variance, and the earlier discussion has shown why this is particularly likely to happen if the number of responses on a recognition test is specified. For the SIM—SPEC condition the guessing correction results in a significant increase of variance (F_{max} (2,23) = 2.65, $p < .02$). Since the within-group variance is a good measure of reliability, it would appear that the guessing correction has lowered reliability, and the purpose and justification of making the correction must be questioned. The answer must involve considerations of validity of measurement as well as reliability of measurement. The purpose of the recognition test is almost always a determination of the knowledge component; and the presence of a guessing component lowers validity, i.e., it reduces the ability of the experimenter to measure what he intends to measure. Thus, scores that are composed of relatively large guessing components in relation to the knowledge component are less valid, and the reduction of the guessing component by a correction factor may increase validity even at the cost of the loss in reliability. This leads to the conclusion that optimum recognition testing must strive to minimize guessing and at the same time deal with the problems that arise when subjects differentially respond to guessing instructions, i.e., use different criteria of certainty in their recognition decisions. Instructing subjects not to guess does not accomplish this objective, since subjects interpret such instructions differentially, and this leads to decreased rather than increased reliability (Frary & Zimmerman, 1970). The use of a specified number of responses with guessing correction and the use of a larger number of foils can contribute toward achieving these objectives.

The purpose of a particular investigation may, of course, dictate the choice of a recognition testing technique. Thus, experiments dealing with signal detection theory are likely to use successive presentation and unspecified number of target items. This technique yields data in a form most suitable for signal detection analysis, and the d' measure is not affected by variability of the decision criterion. Kintsch (1968), Green and Moses (1966), and others have discussed this issue, and it is clear that selection of the appropriate technique must be based upon considerations of validity, not only reliability. It is equally clear, however, that reliability should be a decisive consideration in all those situations in which the choice among techniques is relatively arbitrary, i.e., not clearly determined by the nature of the inquiry.

The present findings show that variance of performance may increase significantly if subjects are allowed to determine the number of target items they select. Thus an investigation of the effects of alcohol, or of any other independent variable, on memory is likely to lead to acceptance of the null hypothesis if the subjects are free to make their own decisions about guessing, and rejection of the null hypothesis if forced guessing is used, assuming the same average effect of the independent variable on recognition performance under the two testing conditions.

THE RELIABILITY OF SUCCESSIVE CRITERIA OF LEARNING

The methods used in the study of learning and memory have been greatly diversified in recent years, but the administration of a succession of training trials terminating when the subject attains a certain performance level remains a standard part of the procedural repertoire of the learning laboratory. Examination of recent issues of the *Journal of Experimental Psychology: Human Learning and Memory* and of the *Journal of Comparative and Physiological Psychology* confirms that the procedure continues to be used with both human and animal subjects in investigations of learning, transfer, and retention. By training subjects to a given criterion level, investigators may establish comparability of performance prior to administering some differential treatment; or they may determine the effect of a treatment condition upon the number of trials needed to reach the criterion level. Thus the effect of alcohol on learning and memory can be investigated by comparing the number of trials needed to reach a criterion level for groups subjected to various dosages of the drug, or subjects who have already been trained to a criterion can be divided into groups who receive various dosages of the drug. The retention performance can then be compared for these groups to determine the effect of the drug treatment. The majority of investigators who have used the trials to criterion design in studies of verbal learning and memory have chosen the first trial on which all of the subjects' responses are correct as the criterion level at which training is terminated. Although this traditional criterion level remains the preferred choice (e.g., Hasher & Johnson, 1975), other criteria also have been used in recent years; e.g., 14 out of 18 items correct (Hasher, Riebman, & Wren, 1976) or 18 out of 20 items correct (Lauer, Streby, & Battig, 1976). The purpose of the present analysis is to establish the variance among individuals associated with the attainment of successive criteria during training and in this way to demonstrate that the power of the experimental design to detect treatment effects varies as a function of the criterion level selected for comparison among the groups.

The data were taken from an investigation in which 60 male and female Ohio Wesleyan University undergraduate students learned a paired-associate list of 12 CVC trigrams by the anticipation method. Thirty of the subjects learned a list of homogeneous difficulty with association values ranging from 55 to 65 (Archer, 1960); the other 30 subjects learned a list of heterogeneous difficulty ranging in association value from 5 to 95. The CVCs were exposed on a memory drum with a 3-second exposure for each stimulus, and an additional 3-second exposure for the stimulus and its paired response. Subjects were given the usual paired-associate learning instructions; an intertrial interval of 9 seconds was used, and training continued to the first trial on which each subject anticipated each of the 12 syllables correctly. Two serial orders of each list were used in alternation on successive trials.

Each subject's record was scored to determine the number of trials required to reach each of 12 successive criteria. Criterion 6, for example, was reached on the first trial on which the subject correctly anticipated any 6 of the 12 CVCs; criterion 12 on the first trial on which all 12 responses were correct. Table 2 shows the results of this analysis for the two groups. Also shown in Table 2 are the mean trial differences between the two groups in reaching successive criteria, and W^2 (Hays, 1973, p. 485), which indicates the portion of the total variance

TABLE 2
Performance Differences During Acquisition

Criteria	Homogeneous list		Heterogeneous list		Mean trial difference	W^2
	Mean trials	SD	Mean trials	SD		
1	2.6	2.9	1.4	1.5	1.2	.18
2	3.7	4.1	2.0	2.3	1.7	.23
3	5.0	5.5	2.9	3.4	2.1	.17
4	6.3	6.8	3.7	4.2	2.6	.19
5	7.8	8.4	4.6	4.9	3.2	.23
6	8.9	9.7	5.8	5.3	3.1	.16
7	11.0	11.6	6.9	7.2	4.1	.23
8	12.3	12.9	8.0	8.4	4.3	.24
9	14.1	14.7	9.6	10.1	4.5	.19
10	16.5	17.1	11.7	12.8	4.8	.10
11	18.0	18.6	14.8	15.4	3.2	.05
12	21.5	22.5	18.4	19.3	3.1	.03

on the dependent variable attributable to the independent variable. The data for each criterion level were subjected to independent analysis of variance, and Figure 1 shows the value of F (1,58) obtained at each criterion level.

It is apparent from inspection of Table 1 that the heterogeneous list was easier than the homogeneous list; i.e., subjects trained with the heterogeneous list reached each successive criterion level in fewer trials than those trained with the homogeneous list. It is further apparent that the mean trial difference between the two groups increases during acquisition, but only up to criterion level 10. The differences actually decline somewhat for the last two criteria. In contrast, the variance associated with individual differences increases at an accelerated rate, particularly for the terminal criterion.

The declining F values obtained for criteria 9 to 12 in Figure 1 are a result of the above relations. With the between-group variance showing little change and the within-group variance increasing, the significance of between-group differences declines. The W^2 index in Table 1 shows the same decline of significance in terms of the portion of variance attributable to the independent variable.

Increased within-group variance at or near terminal criterion levels has been noted previously (Bahrick, 1965, 1967). The sequence of items mastered varies among individuals as a result of subject X item-difficulty interaction. For items of intermediate difficulty, this interaction does not lead to large increases in trial variance among subjects, since there usually are several items of an approximately equal difficulty level selected by various Ss in accordance with their difficulty hierarchy. The contribution to trial variance is likely to be greatest for the last learned, most difficult item, because no other item of approximately

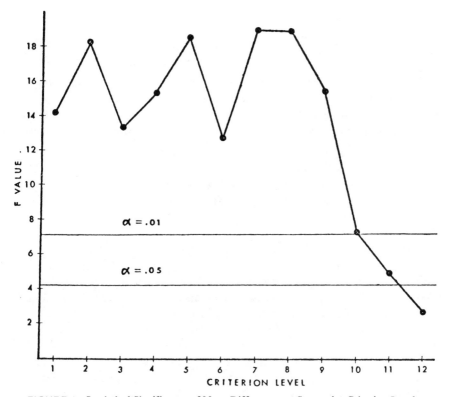

FIGURE 1   Statistical Significance of Mean Differences at Successive Criterion Levels.

comparable difficulty level can be substituted to reduce difficulty variance among subjects.

Declaring the learning rate of two groups to be the same or different on the basis of the trials needed to reach the terminal criterion on a list is comparable to declaring two frequency distributions equivalent or different on the basis of the most extreme scores in the two distributions. Avoidance of the use of extreme anchor points as a basis for comparing distributions has been stressed long ago in other areas of psychology (e.g., the determination of thresholds from distributions of psychophysical responses); but these principles generally have been disregarded in investigations of learning and memory.

Figure 1 shows that the exclusive use of the terminal criterion would lead to the acceptance of the null hypothesis regarding the treatment effect, whereas the use of any other criterion would lead to the rejection of the null hypothesis. Based on the earlier analysis, failure to reject the null hypothesis for the terminal criterion is the result of increased subject X item-difficulty interaction variance. This variance component is rarely of direct interest. It contributes toward unreliability and should be minimized in order to increase the power of the design, i.e., the sensitivity to treatment effects. The use of intermediate criteria is likely to accomplish this result as can be seen in Figure 1. Thus a criterion by criterion analysis of the sort illustrated in the present investigation is likely to provide information on the basis of which more sensitive tests for the effect of an independent variable can be made. Although Melton and his associates (Melton & Irwin, 1940; Melton & von Lackum, 1941) pointed out many years ago the advantages of such criterion—by—criterion analysis in the investigation of learning processes, reliance on terminal criteria has remained a common practice.

VARIANCE INCREMENTS AS INDICANTS
OF SUBJECT X TREATMENT INTERACTION

Subject X treatment interactions have rarely been of direct interest to experimental psychologists. Such interactions usually serve only as the basis of estimating error variance in the assessment of treatment effects. In investigations of drug effects, however, it is not possible to ignore individual differences in response to treatment; and increases of variance among individuals may reveal effects that are not apparent if only mean performance of a group is examined. If the drug acts as a stimulant for some individuals and a depressant for others, the overall mean may reveal no significant treatment effect, because the individual effects offset each other. Cermak's Figure 1 in this volume provides a good illustration of such an interaction. Patients with Korsakoff's syndrome performed more poorly on the cued recall task than on the free recall task, whereas the opposite is observed for the control subjects. Mean performance under cued and free recall is approximately the same for the entire group, and the change in performance characteristic of most subjects would not be revealed unless a separate examination is made of the two subgroups. The presence of such interaction effects can be determined, however, by comparing the variance among subjects before and after treatment; i.e., for the two recall tasks used by Cermak a significant increase of variance is suggestive of interaction. Another basis for identifying the presence of significant subject X treatment interactions is the presence of a negative correlation between the scores obtained by individuals before and after treatment. If the treatment produces opposite effects in two subgroups, or if the treatment affects some individuals but not others, the correlation between scores obtained before and after treatment will diminish or may even be negative if the interaction effect is very strong.

SOME THOUGHTS ABOUT VALIDITY OF MEASUREMENT

Indicants are said to be valid if they measure what they purport to measure. Most textbooks concerned with individual differences (e.g., Anastasi, 1961; Cronbach, 1960) devote an entire chapter to a discussion of the issue of validity of measurement, but the term is unlikely to be found in the subject matter index of textbooks of experimental psychology. The reasons for this contrast are not entirely clear, but among them may be that validity of measurement is more difficult to establish for the experimental psychologist and that measures are often assumed to have face validity. In his thorough discussion of this topic, Melton (1936) pointed out that validity of measurement to the experimental psychologist is basically a question of consistency of measurement and theory. The questions asked about processes not directly observed can be answered only to the extent to which the observed measures reveal these processes. The experimental psychologist generally lacks the type of criterion available to the investigator interested in the validation of a test for the prediction of success in college or success on a job. The task of the experimental psychologist is to establish invariant relations that link response measures of organisms to other conditions. Early in the development of psychological science, progress stalled because the relations between behavioral data and stipulated conscious content could not be verified adequately. The behavioral measures lacked validity for the purpose of answering the questions that were being asked. The observations were compatible with the inferences, but they frequently failed to rule out equally plausible alternative inferences. The resulting impass was temporarily resolved by the behaviorist restriction that excluded questions regarding conscious content and limited psychological inquiry to the investigation of relations between behavioral data and other phenomena subject to direct verification. Within these limited objectives the issue of validity of measurement could be reduced to one of reliability, i.e., reproducibility of the reported relationships. Thus, the relation between the rate of bar pressing of a rat and the amount of alcohol ingested can be established, and the question of validity of the response does not arise so long as the observed relation remains the end product of the inquiry and no additional inferences are drawn about the nature of intervening processes. The radical empiricist position influenced all areas of psychological inquiry, but the injunction against model building and against speculation about the nature of intervening processes did not prevail. The desire to understand how problems are solved, decisions are made, knowledge is organized and retrieved, continues to motivate investigators; and today most of the research concerned with cognitive psychology is again designed to find out more about the nature of processes that are not subject to direct observation (see Segal & Lachman, 1972; Underwood, 1975). Not only questions regarding the nature of imagery but also questions regarding the type of memory search, e.g., self-terminating vs. exhaustive; questions regarding information processing, e.g., from a primary- to a secondary-memory store; questions regarding the retrieval of information, e.g., generation–recognition models; all are answered on the basis of inferences that stipulate intervening processes rendered plausible by the observations. Dependent measures again are being used to answer questions about processes that are not directly observed, and in this context individual measures can no longer be assumed to have face validity. The validity of each indicant depends upon its power to answer the theoretical question that is being asked. It has already been shown that this power is a function of the reliability of the indicant, and in this sense reliability limits validity just as it does in the measurement of individual differences. Beyond the limit imposed by reliability, each response measure reflects somewhat different characteristics; only when these differences are clearly understood and taken into account in the selection of the indicant can high validity of measurement be achieved. Failure to determine the individual characteristics of indicants will limit the progress of cognitive psychology. The programmatic study of interrelations among indicants under a variety of task conditions is therefore a priority.

The data of such research will make it possible to select measures on the basis of their reliability and validity and thus promote the growth of knowledge in the field.

ACKNOWLEDGMENTS

The investigations reported here were supported by Public Health Service Research grant HD 00926-15 from the National Institute of Child Health and Human Development. Appreciation is expressed to Katherine Gharrity and Ruth Hipple Maki for collection and analysis of data.

REFERENCES

Anastasi, A. *Psychological testing*, New York: Macmillan Co., 1961.
Archer, E. J. Re-evaluation of the meaningfulness of all possible CVC trigrams. *Psychological Monographs*, 1960, *74*(10, While No. 497).
Bahrick, H. P. The ebb of retention. *Psychological Review*, 1965, *72*, 60–73.
Bahrick, H. P. Relearning a.id the measurement of retention. *Journal of Verbal Learning and Verbal Behavior*, 1967, *6*, 89–94.
Cronbach, L. J. *Essentials of psychological testing* (2nd ed.). New York: Harper & Row, 1960.
Dixon, W. J., & Massey, F. J., Jr. *Introduction to statistical analysis* (3rd ed.). New York: McGraw-Hill Book Company, 1969.
Frary, R. B., & Zimmerman, D. W. Effect of variation in probability of guessing correctly on reliability of multiple choice tests. *Educational and Psychological Measurement*, 1970, *30*, 595–605.
Green, D. M., & Moses, F. L. On the equivalence of two recognition measures of short-term memory. *Psychological Bulletin*, 1966, *66*, 228–234.
Hasher, L., & Johnson, M. K. Interpretive factors in forgetting. *Journal of Experimental Psychology: Human Learning and Memory*, 1975, *1*, 567–575.
Hasher, L., Riebman, B., & Wren, F. Imagery and the retention of free-recall learning. *Journal of Experimental Psychology: Human Learning and Memory*, 1976, *2*, 172–181.
Hays, W. L. *Statistics for the social sciences* (2nd ed.). New York: Holt, Rinehart & Winston, 1973.
Kintsch, W. An experimental analysis of single stimulus tests and multiple-choice tests of recognition memory. *Journal of Experimental Psychology*, 1968, *76*, 1–6.

Lauer, P. A., Streby, W. J., & Battig, W. F. The effects of alphabetic organization on the acquisition and delayed retention of semantically similar words. *Journal of Experimental Psychology: Human Learning and Memory,* 1976, *2,* 182–189.

Melton, A. W. The methodology of experimental studies of human learning and retention. I. The function of a methodology and the available criteria for evaluating different experimental methods. *Psychological Bulletin,* 1936, *33,* 305–394.

Melton, A. W., & Irwin, J. M. The influence of degree of interpolated learning on retroactive inhibition and the overt transfer of specific responses. *American Journal of Psychology,* 1940, *53,* 173–203.

Melton, A. W., & von Lackum, W. J. Retroactive and proactive inhibition in retention: Evidence for a two-factor theory of retroactive inhibition. *American Journal of Psychology,* 1941, *54,* 157–173.

Segal, E. M., & Lachman, R. Complex behavior or higher mental process: Is there a paradigm shift? *American Psychologist,* 1972, *27,* 46–55.

Thorndike, E. L., & Lorge, I. *The teacher's word book of 30,000 words.* New York: Columbia University, Teachers College Press, 1944.

Underwood, B. J. Individual differences as a crucible in theory construction. *American Psychologist,* 1975, *30,* 128–134.

6
Selective Learning and Forgetting

Geoffrey Keppel
Charles R. Zubrzycki
University of California at Berkeley

Two related puzzles or questions are addressed in this paper. The first is concerned with the fact that very few independent variables that have a profound effect on learning have been shown to influence forgetting. Such important learning variables as meaningfulness and intralist similarity, for example, fail to affect rate of forgetting once learning has been equated in some manner before the start of the retention interval. Since these manipulations were undertaken to test different interference interpretations of forgetting, e.g., that forgetting is due to extra-experimental sources of interference (meaningfulness) or to the recovery of intralist generalization (similarity), the failures to find expected differences in forgetting were damaging to the theories. The second puzzle, which is related to the first, is to explain why and under what circumstances an individual forgets what was originally learned.

No attempt will be made to apply the proposed theory to alcohol research except to mention certain rather obvious points of contact. Although our theory is directed toward the learning and forgetting observed with normal individuals, it still should be able to account for phenomena that are unique to the alcohol area. The conference was a positive step in providing a healthy confrontation of a theory based on normals with data obtained from experiments in which either the ingestion of alcohol is a manipulated variable or in which individuals are studied whose long-term consumption of alcohol has resulted in certain learning and memory deficits.

The context for this discussion will be the paired-associate learning task and the forgetting that is observed when a single list is recalled several hours or days after formal practice has ceased. We will also restrict ourselves to the learning and recall of word pairs, so that we may assume little or no difficulty for subjects in the acquisition of the responses. At this point, however, there is no compelling reason why the theory should not apply to other tasks requiring recall, e.g., serial and free-recall learning. It is not intended to encompass recognition phenomena except when recognition tests are an integral part of the training procedures (cf. Postman and Stark, 1969).

LEARNING AS A SELECTIVE PROCESS

Current conceptualizations of learning assume, with the adult learner at least, that learning is basically a transfer task. Subjects do not learn a list of paired associates from "scratch," but utilize skills and habits acquired over a lifetime of experience with verbal materials. Ease of learning, therefore, is thought to reflect the positive transfer of these skills and habits to the learning task, whereas difficulty of learning is taken to reflect either their zero or negative transfer. For some theorists, the products of acquisition will consist of associations among phonemes, letters, words, phrases, and idea units, and the semantic/linguistic characteristics assumed necessary for effective verbal behavior. Other theorists might add a nonverbal or visual component, with the pairs of words in the learning task being related through their presence in the same image or visual picture (Paivio, 1971). Still others view learning in terms of the nature or level of processing accomplished by the subject during the course of acquisition (e.g., Craik & Lockhart, 1972; Hyde & Jenkins, 1973). We will refer to these associations, mediators, mnemonics, images, and so forth as *encodings* and not worry in this discussion about the exact nature of this obviously important phase of learning.

The encoding process. With these points in mind, we will now consider what happens when a subject first studies one of the pairs included in the list to be learned. It is assumed that during the study interval the word that will serve as the stimulus cue on subsequent tests and the word that is to be given as a response to the stimulus both will suggest a number of potential encodings. The subject's task at this point is to choose an encoding that will be elicited by the stimulus and will lead reliably to the required response. For example, subjects could choose an encoding randomly from the pool of all encodings suggested by the pair at the time of study, or they could "automatically" pick off the first from a hierarchical ordering of the encodings, or they could actively search for a creative way to encode the two members of the pair. The exact basis for the choice and the degree of involvement of the subject are not important for the argument, however.

It is interesting to speculate whether either the stimulus term or the response term dominates the selection of the encoding or whether any such domination is probabilistic and not dictated by one term or the other. When we consider that the subject needs to find some route to the response term in order to be successful on the test trial, we might propose that encodings suggested by the *response term* will dominate the selection process. (If this were true, we might have found the functional basis of so-called "backward" associations between stimuli and responses.) On the other hand, it seems more important for successful performance that the subject discover an encoding that is reliably elicited by the *stimulus* term, since it is the stimulus that must cue the response on the test trials. Direct evidence for the importance of stimulus-related encodings comes from a recent study by Hasher, Griffin, and Johnson (1977). In this experiment, subjects were asked to report the encodings (elaborators) they actually used during learning. These encodings, classified as either stimulus-related or response-related by judges, were given to a new set of subjects to use in learning a list of pairs. Although the nature of the encodings did not influence the speed with which the paired-associate list was acquired, recall scores obtained after a 1-week retention interval clearly favored the subjects who were asked to utilize the stimulus-related encodings.

So far we have been discussing the selection of an encoding for a single pair presented in isolation. In a list, these processes will undoubtedly be influenced to some extent by the presence of the other pairs. For example, the presentation of one pair of words might associatively prime encodings normally elicited by words appearing in other pairs; or a particular linking of two words might influence a subject's selection of encodings for the other pairs in the list. There is no reason to believe, however, that the basic process of encoding and selection will be changed by the particular interpair context of the list.

Interpair interference and selection of encodings.   After the presentation of the pairs, a test trial usually follows in which each stimulus word is presented and the subject attempts to recall the correct response. We will assume that successful performance will be dependent upon the elicitation of the particular encodings that were formed or chosen during study. Unfortunately, these encodings will have been subjected to fairly intense interference before they are given the opportunity to function on the test trial. This interference, which is assumed to occur during the interval between the study and eventual test of any given pair, results from the subsequent presentation of other pairs for study and for test (Tulving & Arbuckle, 1963). A pair in a 10-pair list, for example, which is presented in the 4th position on the study trial and in the 9th position on the test trial, will have had 6 pairs presented for study and 8 pairs presented for test before it is finally tested for recall. The deleterious effect of presenting other pairs or stimuli during the interval between the study and test of a particular pair represents a retroactive source of interpair interference. If we add to this interference the potential proactive source of interference from pairs that have been presented previously on the study trial, we can expect considerable amounts of forgetting to occur between the study and test portions of the trial.[1] This retention loss is important, however, since it is assumed to play a critical role in the total learning process. To be more specific, we will assume that this intratrial forgetting functions as a *selective filter* through which will pass only those encodings that can successfully survive the interpair interference generated in the list.

Consider next what happens on the second study trial. Encodings that successfully supported recall on the first test trial may no longer be effective due to the potential operation of additional interpair interference produced by the interpolation of other pairs for test on the test trial and for study on the second study trial. (For example, a pair in a 10-pair list that was tested in the 4th position on the first test trial and presented in the 3rd position on the second study trial will have been subjected to the interpolation of 6 pairs for test and 2 pairs for study during the test–study interval for that particular pair.) Any loss of previously successful encodings during this interval will simply result in a more selective filtering of the encodings. For encodings that were not elicited on the first test trial, it is unlikely that they will become available after the test because of the additional interpair interference generated during the test–study interval.

Upon the presentation of each pair for study on this new study trial, subjects will attempt to maintain those encodings that were successful previously. This may consist of an "old-fashioned" strengthening or perhaps a "layering" of additional encodings. On the other hand, when subjects are confronted with a pair that was not recalled successfully or whose encoding was lost through the interference generated during the test–study interval, they will cast about for an encoding that this time will prove to be resistant to interpair interference. Subjects might even choose to use previously unsuccessful encodings on subsequent trials. Such encoding persistence (Greeno, James & DaPolito, 1971) would not be considered the optimal strategy for subjects to use, however. Instead, it is assumed that subjects will choose a different encoding from the pool of potential encodings. It is not important whether this sampling is random or calculated, whether it occurs with or without replacement, or whether the pool of encodings for any given pair changes from trial to trial. What is critical, however, is the use of new encodings for pairs that failed to be recalled on the previous test trial.

Interpair interference will again operate to identify successful encodings, and the cycle will begin again. Additional sets of study and test trials, which we can now call selection cycles, will be administered until the subject finds a sufficient

---

[1] Tulving (1964) discusses in detail the role of intratrial forgetting in multiple trial–free recall.

number of successful encodings to attain the level of performance set by the experimenter.

Other tasks and learning variables. Although this discussion has focused on paired-associate learning, there is no reason why the theory cannot be applied to other learning tasks. In fact, Tulving (1964) has proposed a similar filtering mechanism to account for certain phenomena in free-recall learning. Specifically, words that survive subsequent study and recall of other words become incorporated into an organization of "successful" words, an organization that is continually evolving and increasing in size with practice. Our theory would suggest that this higher-order organization is an example of the "successful encoding" assumed for paired associates that are recalled after having been submitted to considerable amounts of interpair interference. Although with paired associates the encodings for different pairs will tend to be independent from one another, this would appear not to be the case in free-recall learning. In free recall, words become interdependent and organized so that encodings of groups of words will reflect sizable overlap when compared with paired associates. In any case, the two processes seem to be compatible.

Any account of the acquisition process must provide some explanation of how variables that influence speed of learning operate. In the present theory, there are two factors that might ultimately influence speed of learning. The first of these involves processes operating on the speed with which successful encodings can be found on the study trial. It may be that it is this aspect of learning that is largely responsible for the effect of stimulus meaningfulness on learning, where stimuli of low meaningfulness would tend to elicit weak and unreliable encodings (cf. Martin, 1968). The second factor involves processes operating during the interval between study and test, i.e., the interference generated by the interpolation of other pairs for study and other stimuli for test. It may be that this input/output interference is largely responsible for the negative effect of intralist similarity on learning, where pairs of high similarity produce large amounts of interpair interference due to the overlap of physical or semantic features among the pairs in the list. Both factors — encoding selection and interpair interference — may be needed to account for the operation of other variables, e.g., differences between slow and fast subjects, or the general improvement in performance when subjects learn a series of unrelated lists (learning-to-learn transfer).

Summary. Acquisition is viewed as the selection and testing of tentative encodings, with interpair interference providing the mechanism by which unstable, unreliable, or inappropriate encodings are eliminated and successful ones are retained. Said another way, the filtering out of encodings that cannot survive the interference generated by the other pairs in the list results in the attainment of a set of stimulus—response encodings that are *compatible* with one another.

AN EXPERIMENTAL ANALOGUE

One way to study the selective-learning process proposed in this paper would be to obtain a normative collection of possible encodings for each pair in the list and then to trace their selection and their fate during the course of acquisition. An analogue of this selection process is provided by some data collected during the one-trial learning controversy of the early 1960s. For reasons that will not be discussed, Rock (1957) introduced a condition in which pairs recalled correctly on any given test trial were retained in the list for the next study trial; pairs that were not recalled or were recalled incorrectly were replaced by new pairs drawn randomly from a large pool of pairs from which the original study list was also randomly drawn. If it is assumed that the pairs in the pool varied in difficulty, the dropout procedure should result in the retention of the easier pairs and the elimination of the more difficult pairs from the learning task. Replacement with new pairs and the subsequent dropping of pairs missed would lead to a continued selection of easy pairs in the list being learned. Underwood, Rehula, and Keppel (1962) showed clear selection of easy pairs with this procedure from a pool of pairs of known differences in difficulty. This selection process renders the dropout procedure useless for the one-trial learning question, but it does provide evidence for the operation of a selective filter during paried-associate learning.

Admittedly, the selection observed with the Rock dropout condition is not the same as that proposed here for standard paired-associate learning. With the Rock procedure, the failure of a pair to be recalled on a test for whatever reason results in the elimination of this pair from the learning task. In the standard condition upon which our theory is based, all pairs are retained on successive trials; but the particular *encodings* of missed pairs are lost and are presumably replaced by new ones. With the former procedure, then, there is the random replacement of pairs missed *and* the selection of an encoding of these replacements by the subjects. With the latter procedure, the pairs do not change and the selection is only from pools of possible encodings for each individual pair. On the other hand, the evidence obtained from the dropout procedure does support the general logic of the selective-learning notion.

Experiments could be designed to study the selection of successful encodings more directly. For example, subjects at different stages of practice could be asked to report their encodings for each pair in the list. Then, in a manner introduced by Hasher and Johnson (1975), new groups of subjects would be asked to use these encodings to learn the list. Recall tests after a long retention interval should show considerable forgetting when the subjects are asked to use the relatively unfiltered encodings obtained on the initial learning trials and greatly reduced forgetting when the subjects use the highly filtered encodings obtained at higher stages of learning. The major drawback of this procedure is its reliance on the presence of strong normative agreement among subjects in the rejection and selection of specific encodings of the different pairs in the list. Since a positive outcome for the theory is not possible without a reasonable amount of normative agreement and, for that matter, a willingness of subjects to use the particular encodings they have been supplied, any negative outcome must be viewed with a certain amount of caution. A positive outcome, of course, represents convincing support for the theory.

FORGETTING AND INTERPAIR COMPATIBILITY

The learning process we have been considering is based on a principle of "natural selection," the final result of which is the evolution of a set of encodings that have high "survival value" in the verbal environment of the list being learned. At the end of learning, the subject has acquired a set of encodings that are mutually compatible in the sense that they can coexist in the subject's memory and can be retrieved. We will assume that interpair compatibility varies as a function of a subject's stage of practice on the list and that the degree of compatibility can be indexed by the recall performance achieved on any given test trial. We will assume further that if two different groups learning either different sets of material or the same list under different treatments are taken to the same performance criterion, e.g., one perfect recitation, that they will be roughly equated in terms of interpair compatibility. Said another way, training continues until a sufficient amount of interpair compatibility is attained in order to support the required recall performance.

We can now accommodate the numerous failures to find differential forgetting as a function of variables that influence learning by assuming that forgetting and interpair compatibility are inversely related, i.e., the greater the interpair compatibility, the less the forgetting. This also implies, of course, that forgetting will be the same whenever different treatment groups achieve the same degree of interpair compatibility at the end of training. If it is any consolation to theorists who have predicted differences in forgetting, one could argue that the expected differential forgetting occurred during *learning* – during the interval between study and test. That is, if we were able to measure precisely the amount of forgetting occurring between study and test on any given trial for two groups treated differently, we might find greater losses for the more difficult condition.[2] A list containing highly similar pairs, for example, might show greater intratrial forgetting than will a list of dissimilar pairs. This differential is not allowed to remain, however, since subjects are usually forced to continue training until the differential intratrial forgetting no longer occurs – namely, at

---

[2] It is possible that subjects may fail to establish encodings for certain pairs during the study interval, in which case an inability to recall the response could not be attributable to intratrial forgetting but rather to encoding failure.

the point where equal interpair compatibility is achieved. Differential forgetting is not observed over the considerably longer retention interval, because the subject has finally found encodings that are resistant to the sort of interpair interference generated by a list of highly similar pairs.

The idea that subjects establish encodings that resist or compensate for differences in interpair interference has been expressed by others. Battig (1966, 1968), for example, has suggested that a list generating high interpair interference will bring into play higher-order learning processes such as interpair grouping, which will serve as a source of facilitation in subsequent retention. He speculates that theories that have predicted differential forgetting from extralist sources, e.g., linguistic sources of interference proposed by Underwood and Postman (1960), have failed to find these differences because of the compensating facilitation from the differential engagement of paired-associate learning processes required to overcome interpair interference.[3] The difference between Battig's speculations and ours is that he favors the view that major learning variables have not influenced forgetting because of an inverse relationship between intratask interference and extratask sources of interference operating over the retention interval. We have assumed, however, that there are no extratask sources of interference that differentially operate on lists varying in meaningfulness or similarity.

The notions presented so far explain why variables such as meaningfulness and similarity fail to affect rate of long-term forgetting. To have any generality, the selective-learning hypothesis must be able to explain why certain other variables *do* influence forgetting. We will consider these explanations briefly.

Degree of learning.   One variable that is consistently found to affect forgetting is degree of learning: the higher the degree of learning, the less the forgetting (e.g., Underwood & Keppel, 1963). Since we have indicated that degree of learning and degree of interpair compatibility are correlated, we should say something about the relationship between these two concepts. Degree of learning has been conceptualized in terms of associative strength and in terms of number of memory attributes (Underwood, 1969). The present conceptualization, when reduced to the level of an individual paired associate, can easily incorporate current theoretical descriptions of degree of learning. What distinguishes interpair compatibility from degree of learning is the notion of the establishment of associations that can coexist in memory and a specification of how the acquisition process takes place.

Distributed practice.   A variable introduced during learning that affects forgetting is distributed practice. Underwood and his associates originally discovered that interpolating rests or temporal spaces between acquisition trials would

---

[3] A similar notion has been proposed by Joinson and Runquist (1968).

reduce the amount of forgetting. These initial studies indicated that the effect was found only under conditions of high associative interference from lists learned previously in the laboratory (Underwood, Keppel & Schulz, 1962; Underwood & Schulz, 1961). In these experiments, the amount of spacing varied from 1 to 3 minutes. Subsequently, Keppel (1964) found that extremely long spacing intervals, i.e., 24 hours between successive pairs of trials, essentially eliminated the negative effect of the prior lists (proactive inhibition). These findings were interpreted in terms of an interference theory that assumed that the distribution intervals allowed the more effective extinction of previously learned interlist associations and, consequently, reduced interlist competition at the time of recall.

A later study (Keppel, 1967) cast serious doubt on this explanation. In Experiment III of that study, the retention of a single list of paired associates that was learned by massed practice (i.e., 8 training trials with 4 seconds between successive trials), was compared with the retention of the same list learned by distributed practice (i.e., a 24-hour interval between successive pairs of trials). Following the termination of learning, subjects in the two training conditions were tested for final recall after 1 day or after 8 days. After 1 day, the massed subjects retained 81% of what they had learned, whereas the distributed subjects retained 95%. After 8 days, the massed subjects retained 29%, and the distributed subjects retained 81%.

The spacing effect was interpreted in terms of a selective-learning process that is consistent with the theoretical ideas discussed in this paper. More specifically, the long spacing intervals administered during acquisition allow the encodings selected during the study intervals to be filtered through the same sorts of factors that are presumed to operate over the retention interval, which will be introduced after the training is finally completed. Encodings that survive these distribution intervals will have been selected on the basis of the kinds of cues that will be present on the *final retention test* — either 1 or 8 days following learning — and thus, will result in a close correspondence between the encodings acquired during learning and those aroused at the final recall.

Proactive inhibition. If subjects are asked to learn a series of unrelated paired-associate lists, recall declines steadily as a function of the number of lists previously learned and recalled in the laboratory (Keppel, Postman, & Zavortink, 1968). Current interpretations of this proactive effect of previously learned material stress the loss of the response set and of the discriminability of the list last learned (Postman & Keppel, in press). Though not denying the operation of these mechanisms at the time of recall, the present theory would maintain that the selection of encodings during acquisition was on the basis of success in surviving the interpair interference present during *learning* and not necessarily on the basis of *interlist* or *between-list* interference. Thus, the selection is appropriate for the interference operating during *acquisition,* when interlist mechanisms are probably operating at a minimum, but not for the interlist interference that will be present at the time of recall.

Theoretically, proactive inhibition should be greatly reduced or even eliminated if interlist interference can be introduced *during acquisition* so that encodings can be filtered through the sorts of interference that will be critical *on the retention test*. We have already considered one way by which this can be accomplished, namely, through the introduction of long intertrial intervals in learning. These intervals allow interlist factors to operate on the encodings currently in use by the subject and to leave as active only encodings that are resistant to the form of interference peculiar to the multiple-list situation. The effectiveness of such intervals has been reported in an experiment by Keppel (1964) in which subjects recalled the fourth in a series of associatively related lists (same stimuli, but different responses in the four lists) following either massed practice (minimal intervals between trials) or distributed practice (24 hours between pairs of trials). After 1 day, retention was 16% for the massed subjects and 89% for the distributed subjects; after 8 days, retention was 3% and 72%, respectively. Although it can be shown that massive amounts of proactive inhibition were present in this experiment, the distributed subjects seem to be immune to its negative effects. A comparison with a subsequent study (Keppel, 1967), in which a single list was learned and recalled, tends to support this conclusion. More specifically, retention scores for the distributed subjects in this latter study were 95% and 81% after 1 and 8 days, respectively, so that proactive inhibition (single-list retention minus fourth-list retention) was only minimal, namely, 6% and 9%, respectively.

These results are only suggestive, of course, and further studies are needed to implicate directly the selective-learning mechanism. One such investigation would require the collection of encodings from subjects learning a single list or a fourth list by either massed or distributed practice and then the supply of these encodings to new subjects learning these lists by massed practice. Assuming normative agreement, it would be expected that subjects receiving encodings from massed subjects will show more forgetting and greater proactive inhibition than subjects receiving the encodings obtained from distributed subjects.

SELECTIVE LEARNING AND FORGETTING

Up to this point, we have been discussing why certain variables do or do not influence forgetting and have left unanswered why forgetting occurs no matter what level of interlist compatibility has been achieved at the end of learning.

A Cause of Forgetting

The acquisition process, consisting of the selection of encodings of the stimulus and response terms and the filtering out of encodings that are unable to survive the verbal environment of that particular list, has been described already in considerable detail. Recall performance, whether during acquisition or following a retention interval, is dependent upon the arousal of the encodings that were selected during study. If we are talking about recall performance during learning, we are referring to the encodings that are selected or maintained on the immediately preceding study trial. If we are talking about recall performance after a retention interval, we are referring to the encodings established by the end of learning. Forgetting will occur if these encodings fail to be elicited on the retention test.

A close experimental analogue of this model of forgetting is the paradigm introduced by Tulving and Osler (1968). In their experiment, some subjects were provided with word cues with which they were to associate a set of to-be-recalled words; other subjects were given no such cues. At recall, subjects attempted to recall these words either with or without the cues provided during study or with an entirely new set of cues. The important finding for our purposes was that recall was higher when the cue conditions in study and test were the same than when the cue conditions were different.

The problem of extending the findings of Tulving and Osler to the forgetting paradigm is the fact that in the standard paired-associate experiment the encodings and cues utilized by the subject during learning are not explicit. Consequently, one can only state as an article of faith that the forgetting of an individual pair was due to a failure to arouse the appropriate encoding at recall. A procedure developed by Montague, Adams, and Kiess (1966) might possibly provide a means for studying this critical aspect of the present theory. Briefly, they asked subjects to report any encodings they had formed during the single study period given each pair of nonsense syllables. On a retention test 24 hours later, subjects were asked to recall the correct response and, if possible, the encoding as well. They found better performance when subjects were able to recall the encoding formed during learning than when they could not do so. Unfortunately, there is a confounding of degree of learning and whether or not a subject reported an encoding after pair presentation, but the use of subject reports concerning the utilization of encodings during learning and at recall might shed some light on acquisition as well as on forgetting.

Reasons for the Elicitation of Inappropriate Encodings

Now that we have identified a major reason why we forget, namely, a failure to elicit the encodings established during learning at the time of recall, we have left still unanswered the question of why the proper encodings are not aroused. Several possibilities will be considered.

Recovery of dominant encodings. A first possibility is suggested by the acquisition process itself. We assumed that each verbal unit functioning as a stimulus or as a response in a paired-associate list has its own hierarchy of encodings. It is from this pool of encodings that the subject selects candidates to be tried on the next test trial. We will assume that the encodings highest or most dominant in the hierarchies of the stimulus and response terms are not always the ones eventually retained by the subject at the end of learning. If over the retention interval the encodings return to their original hierarchical arrangement, the appropriate encoding will not be aroused by the stimulus cue at the time of recall, and forgetting will occur.[4]

Evidence for the recovery of free-association hierarchies after a shift has been induced experimentally has been reported in the literature. Briggs (1954), for example, found a drop in free-association responding to words after they served as stimuli in two paired-associate lists and a recovery in free-association responding during a retention interval introduced following the termination of learning. E. A. Bilodeau (e.g., 1967) has studied changes in free-association strength more directly by assessing the effects of a number of manipulations on the recall of initially strong free associates. In a different sort of paradigm, Maltzman and his associates have studied the effects of forcing subjects to give a series of free associations to the same set of stimulus words. They consistently have found a decrease in normative responding as subjects continue to give associates; and in one experiment, they reported a recovery of normative responding over a 48-hour period (Maltzman, Simon, Raskin, & Licht, 1960, Experiment 5).

Given the possibility of the recovery of stronger free associates over a retention interval following the acquisition of a weaker or less dominant one, we would expect to find greater forgetting when paired associates consist of low-probability free associates than when they consist of high-probability free associates. Interestingly, such findings have been reported both for recall (e.g., Postman, Fraser, & Burns, 1968) and for recognition (Turnage, 1963). Although not all attempts to show forgetting as a function of free-association strength have been successful (cf. Keppel, 1968, 1972), the occasional report of positive outcomes offers encouragement to the speculation that at least one source of forgetting is the recovery of dominant encodings.

The results of these various studies provide support for mechanisms that are thought to operate during the learning and retention of paired associates. If a similar process is involved in the elicitation and selection of paired-associate encodings as appears to be involved with free associates, forgetting will certainly be the expected result.

Changes in the subject. A second potential contributor to the arousal of inappropriate encodings at recall is the fact that the subject has changed over the retention interval and that his or her psychological and physiological environ-

---

[4] This mechanism is also related to Martin's (1968) conceptualization of encoding variability. He proposed that any given stimulus term may be responded to (i.e., encoded) in a number of ways, the probability of any particular encoding being dependent upon its probability density over the entire set of possible encodings for that stimulus. This assumed instability of stimulus encodings may provide sufficient variability in the encodings elicited at recall to produce the 10 to 20 percent forgetting generally observed over a 24-hour period. (See Keppel (1972) for a detailed discussion of this possibility.)

ments are somewhat different than they were at the time of learning. When the subjects return to the laboratory, they will have lived through experiences that are different from those they experienced before the start of the learning session. They will have different anticipations, expectations, moods, attitudes, and motivations when they return for the delayed memory test. If any of these psychological changes adversely affects the elicitation of appropriate encodings at recall, forgetting will occur. Evidence in support of this expectation has been reported by Weingartner and Murphy (1974) who found that changes in a subject's mood between learning and recall resulted in lowered retention performance.

Some attempts at manipulating a subject's physiological state during learning and recall also have been reported. One interesting finding, which should be investigated further, was reported by Rand and Wapner (1967). Briefly, they varied postural cues by requiring subjects to learn a serial list of nonsense syllables in either an erect or a supine position and to relearn the list 15 minutes later in either the same or changed body position. Relearning (to one perfect recitation) was accomplished significantly faster when the learning—relearning postures were congruent than when they were not.

The state-dependent manipulations provide another means for determining the role of a match or mismatch of physiological states induced by the differential administration of drugs. With humans, most of this research has used alcohol as a way of efficiently (and pleasantly) changing a sober person's internal state. State dependency is considered demonstrated when subjects tested in the same drug state (drug—drug and placebo—placebo) show better retention performance than do subjects tested in a changed drug state (drug—placebo and placebo—drug). We will not review this literature, since the topic is discussed and explored by Eich (this volume).

Eich's analysis does reveal that state-dependent effects can be found in humans. Moreover, he suggests that they are found more successfully with tasks that require "the processing and utilization of order information [p. 147]." Included among such tasks are tasks that require sequence reproduction (e.g., serial recall and memory for the sequence in which a series of lights flash) and single-trial free recall. An alternative possibility, which was originally suggested by Peterson (1976) and which is equally well supported by the data, is that state-dependent effects are most easily demonstrated with tasks in which subjects must provide their own retrieval cues rather than having relevant cues provided at recall by the experimenter.[5] We favor this

---

[5] Under this method of classification, the free-recall task certainly would be considered an example of the first category and the paired-associate task a clear example of the second category. Serial recall, on the other hand, is difficult to classify, although the fact that the task does force subjects to generate their own specific cues, whether temporal, positional, or associational, tends to suggest that the first category is a more appropriate classification than the second.

alternative interpretation, since our theory would expect greater state-dependency effects with tasks in which subjects must rely more on internal cues than with tasks in which subjects can use the explicit recall cues provided by the experimenter. In any case, the speculation that state-dependency effects are task specific is important for this general research area, as these findings will help to pinpoint the nature of the memory deficits observed when the learning–recall drug states are incongruent.

Physiological changes of a different sort may also be present. For instance, the subject might be functioning under different drive states than were present during learning. It is even possible that changes due to variations in basic biological rhythms may subtly affect a subject's reaction to verbal stimuli on the retention test.[6] In fact, periodic variations in retention have been observed with animals. Holloway and Wansley (1973), for example, tested rats for the retention of a 1-trial, passive-avoidance task from 15 minutes to 72 hours. Animals tested at successive 12-hour intervals demonstrated "perfect or near-perfect" retention, whereas animals tested 6 hours after training and at successive 12-hour intervals demonstrated relatively poor retention. There was also the suggestion of a 24-hour cycle superimposed over the shorter one.

Circadian fluctuations in human performance have been well documented (Colquhoun, 1971; Posner, 1975). Blake (1971) reports that memory span for digits declines systematically during the day. If circadian changes in long-term memory can be firmly established with humans, as they have with lower animals, we may have identified an important source of forgetting. Our theory suggests that the locus of any circadian effect will be the elicitation of inappropriate encodings at recall. Assuming that individuals have biological cycles of different lengths, and that subjects are asked to learn and recall at different times during the day, the result would be a gradually declining retention function when the data from different subjects, who are trained and tested at different times and who have circadian cycles of different lengths, are averaged together to produce an overall function. If individuals have cycles longer or shorter than 24 hours, retention intervals of long duration will result in an increasing deviation of learning and testing physiological states as each day passes. (Eventually a subject's cycle will "catch up" with the 24-hour clock of the experimenter, and retention performance should improve!) Although much of this argument may turn out to be wild speculation, the chance of finding "memory cycles" in humans is an extremely interesting possibility.

Changes in the testing environment.   Finally, it is possible that changes in the environment of the testing situation may affect the arousal of appropriate encodings at recall. The classical study by I. McD. Bilodeau and Schlosberg

---

[6] We wish to thank Professor Irving Zucker for originally suggesting this possibility and Ms. Elizabeth Kruesi for sharing with us a review of the literature.

(1951) varied the experimental context in which a second interfering list was learned. They found that retroactive inhibition (reduced recall of the first list as the result of learning the second list) was reduced when the second list was learned in an experimental setting that was greatly changed from that in which the critical first list was learned.[7] Of greater relevance to our theory are studies in which the change-of-context manipulation is imposed on the learning and recall of a given list. In its basic form the design consists of two conditions, one in which subjects learn and recall in the same experimental context and one in which they learn and recall in different experimental contexts. Greenspoon and Ranyard (1957) included these two conditions and found poorer recall of a serial list when the learning—recall contexts were changed than when they were unchanged. These and other similar findings were obtained with the retroactive-inhibition paradigm, however. What we need are studies manipulating the learning—recall context of a *single* list.

We have attempted to find such context-change effects in both the single-list and retroactive-inhibition designs, but with no success. In one study, for example, subjects learned a paired-associate list to a criterion of 9/12 correct responses on one trial and then were tested for recall after either 18 minutes or 24 hours in either the same experimental room or in a discriminably different room. Results showed no effect of context change after either retention interval. We also failed to obtain the classical context effects in the retroactive-inhibition portion of the experiment.[8]

In spite of our negative findings, there is some positive evidence to report. We have already mentioned the study by Rand and Wapner (1967) in which a change in the subject's *internal* environmental context (same or different body position) slowed down the relearning of a serial list. An experiment by Godden and Baddeley (1975) studied the effect of context change in a rather dramatic (and severe) manipulation of the learning—recall environment. Briefly, divers learned a list of words above or below the surface of a lake in Scotland. The words studied in the two environments were recalled either above water or under water by the method of free recall. They found sizable effects of context change, namely, poorer recall when the learning—recall context was different than when it was the same.

Manipulations that have been successful in producing context-dependent effects are much more severe than the small and subtle changes that occur in the usual retention study. What we might call "unnatural" context manipulations,

---

[7] These findings have been questioned by Strand (1970), who demonstrated that an equivalent reduction in interference could be obtained by taking the subject for a walk and returning to the *same* experimental room as was found by going instead to a *different* room.

[8] Subsequent experiments conducted in our laboratory have shown that changing the learning context of a second list while holding constant the learning—recall context of the first list does significantly reduce retroactive inhibition for *serial lists* even when a control for disruption is introduced.

e.g., changes in learning environments (different rooms, on land or under water) or in body position, are still valuable, however, in that they test the limits of a theoretical mechanism or process. That is, if context effects can *not* be demonstrated with these sorts of manipulations, then the theory is in trouble. Since context effects *can* be shown, we can use these manipulations to study in detail the operation of the proposed theoretical mechanisms.

Nonspecific Interference

A final possible source of forgetting is what has been called nonspecific interference. Some years ago, Keppel (1968) proposed that a subject's verbal activity during the retention interval is responsible for forgetting. This mechanism, which is retroactive in nature, was assumed to be nonspecific, operating with no selectivity on materials learned in the laboratory. Although recent experiments have not been favorable (cf. Keppel, 1972), they also have not duplicated the conditions of interpolation that are assumed to occur daily during the subject's waking (and perhaps dreaming) life. Moreover, these experiments have not examined the possibility that this nonspecific interference may have its effect by changing and shifting the hierarchies of encodings associated with the stimulus and response terms, the result of which would also be a failure of recall.

Summary

Our theory proposes that forgetting is due to the elicitation of inappropriate encodings at the time of recall. In this section, we have listed a number of factors that might be responsible for recall failure. Obviously, it is not possible to determine at this time whether the operation of these factors will account for all of the forgetting observed in the standard retention study, or whether our explanation of these findings in terms of the elicitation of inappropriate encodings is correct. It should be remembered, however, that we do not have to account for especially large retention losses. (No more than 20% retention loss is observed over 24 hours for single lists learned to a reasonable criterion of mastery.) Thus, any of these potential factors or any combination of them might trigger off a sufficient number of inappropriate encodings on the retention test to account for whatever forgetting is observed. In addition, we should not overlook the possibility that just one recall failure might disrupt the associative context of the list, i.e., the interpair compatibility, and magnify the retention loss. This sort of "snowball" effect might be observed in paired-associate learning when stimulus or response terms are interrelated, in serial learning when an item is missed at the beginning of the list, or in a free-recall task when a word is lost that serves as a retrieval cue for a "subjective unit" consisting of a number of words.

STATE-DEPENDENT LEARNING: A METHODOLOGICAL NOTE

In searching for support for our theory in the state-dependency literature, we encountered some critical interpretive problems based on design. These design issues have plagued our own research area in verbal learning, and we want to share our concerns with the participants at the conference.

Overton (1974) has also criticized the state-dependency paradigm, arguing that the confounding of drug-related processes and the inability of statistics to disentangle these component processes seriously disputes the efficacy of this paradigm. His criticisms are conceptual in nature, specifying processes such as novelty effects and performance decrements that may operate together to produce any given set of data, even the typical state-dependency results. We leave to other participants of the conference the task of dealing with these interactions of processes, since they are unique to drug research.

Equation of Degree of Learning

Basically, a state-dependent learning study, or any retention experiment for that matter, consists of two stages — namely, acquisition and retention. With the types of designs with which we are dealing, in which different treatments are administered during both stages, differences in performance resulting from manipulations during acquisition necessarily cloud the interpretation of differences observed at recall. More specifically, any retention differences may be due either to the Day 1 manipulation per se (acquisition drug state), to any differences in *learning* resulting from the Day 1 manipulation, to the Day 2 manipulation, or to the interactions of any of these components.

The degree-of-learning issue is by far the most critical aspect of a retention experiment. Suppose we start an experiment in which the same number of training trials is administered to a faster learning group (control in an alcohol study) and to a slower learning group (alcohol group). Let us assume that the control group recalls 5 items more than the alcohol group immediately following learning and that this difference increases to 7 items 24 hours later. Analyses indicate that the Day 2 difference is greater than the Day 1 difference. Is it safe to conclude that the alcohol group shows greater forgetting than the control group, based on the Day 1 treatment? Definitely not, since we have no way of ascertaining whether with these particular materials and with this particular manipulation forgetting is faster because of the difference in treatment or because of the lower degree of learning. We clearly have no common baseline from which to measure differential forgetting for the two groups.

Two general techniques are available to equate degree of learning when differences in learning rate are probable. The first involves administering a differential number of trials to each group, but holding constant the number of trials given to the subjects in any one group.[9] For example, all subjects in a drug group might receive 10 training trials whereas control subjects might receive only 7 trials. The trials needed by the two groups to achieve equivalent degrees of learning would have been obtained through pilot work. An alternative procedure would be to vary the exposure durations for the two groups – 4 seconds per item for the alcohol subjects, for example, and 2 seconds for the control subjects – although this method is not as common as the former. Again, pilot work would have to be conducted to determine the exact combination of exposure times that will achieve an equation of degree of learning.[10]

There are several difficulties with this particular solution to the problem. First, the method is inefficient in the sense that pilot work must be conducted in order to find the adjustment combinations necessary to equate degree of learning. Second, it must be realized that varying either trials or exposure durations introduces a new confounding into the experiment, namely, more trials or longer durations for the alcohol group. On the other hand, it appears that a confounding of trials with treatments is not as pernicious as the confounding of degree of learning with treatments, since we can show that trials per se are not an important factor in forgetting (Keppel, Postman, & Zavortink, 1968, pp. 795–796). Finally, subjects within any group will vary widely in the degree of learning they individually achieve, though the groups themselves will not vary. A large amount of within-group variability may decrease the likelihood of finding significant retention differences but the problem can be solved most easily by increasing sample size.

The second method insures that all subjects will have a common baseline from which to measure forgetting, since each subject is taken to a common criterion of performance, e.g., 9 out of 12 correct responses on a single trial. This technique is more efficient than the first, since a pilot study is no longer required. In addition, intersubject variability in degree of learning is reduced, increasing the sensitivity of the retention test. An even closer matching of subjects can be achieved through the use of an adjusted-learning task (Amster, Keppel, & Meyer, 1970).

Both methods of equating degree of learning are effective when the speed of acquisition does not vary greatly between groups, but problems arise when there is a great disparity. Underwood (1964) discusses in detail the problem of overshooting the criterion by the faster learning groups. If one were to extrapolate the learning curves of fast and slow learning groups, one would find that faster learners would be expected to recall more on the next trial than the slower subjects. This is due to the greater slope of the acquisition curve for the fast

---

[9] Postman, Fraser, and Burns (1968) report an experiment in which this technique was effectively employed.
[10] Shuell and Keppel (1970) provide an example of this sort of adjustment.

subjects, and the projection is essential in order to account for the learning that will occur on the final acquisition trial.

Obversely, the slower learners will have greatly overlearned a subset of the items, which should then be more resistant to forgetting. Though researchers have attempted to circumvent this problem by dropping out an item from the presentation list once it is mastered, this technique creates additional problems (Amster et al., 1970; Underwood, 1954). This overlearning can be moderated, however, by choosing a criterion that is short of 1 perfect recitation; for example, 9 out of 12 correct responses. Since it is the most difficult items that are learned last and that greatly increase the number of trials needed to attain criterion, a lower criterion will decrease the number of overlearning trials that the easy items receive. Also, a high criterion may decrease the sensitivity of the immediate test due to ceiling effects, especially when subjects reach criterion quickly (Underwood, 1964). (Bahrick, this volume, presents some data showing the effects that a high criterion can have on detecting learning differences as well.)

To insure that degree of learning is equivalent, researchers now assess retention shortly following learning. But since learning does occur on this test trial, new groups of subjects are needed to assess delayed recall. Thus, we would visualize a state-dependency experiment as consisting of six independent groups: two groups to assess the degree of learning of the drug and control manipulations, in addition to the four usual state-dependency groups. Only if analyses reveal no immediate-group differences can we be assured that degree of learning has been equated and only then can we interpret the forgetting of the state-dependency groups.

A frequently used forgetting paradigm, especially for recognition memory, is one in which a single list is presented for study and not tested until a day or so later. Based on our previous analysis, one can see that if any differences in acquisition are expected, this paradigm can say nothing about interpreting any forgetting differences that may be observed. That is, having no immediate test with which to assess the level of initial acquisition (learning), one can only conclude that degree-of-learning differences will contribute to any retention effect.

Comparison of Retention Tests

Researchers of state dependency have specified their theories well enough to study other learning paradigms, such as recognition and cuing tests, and degree of learning is critical here, too. Bahrick (1964) makes the point that degree of learning must be equated with respect to the type of test with which retention will finally be assessed. Bahrick argues that the sensitivity of any retention measure is a constantly changing function of the threshold of individual items for that particular retention measure. Thus, if subjects learn a list under free-recall procedures, they may show no forgetting even days later when tested by recognition, because the individual items are too far above the threshold of forgetting for a recognition test. The list simply has been learned too well with regard to recognition to demonstrate forgetting.

The easiest method for equating degree of learning is to use the same type of test during both the test trials administered in learning and the test trials administered after the retention interval. Again, only an immediate retention test will assure that degree of learning is properly equated in both cuing and recognition paradigms.

Multiple-Task Studies

In our review of the state-dependency literature, we found studies in which more than one learning task was administered during the first stage of the experiment. Retention for these different tasks was assessed during the second stage. Although such a procedure provides information on more than one training task, the findings are probably not capable of interpretation. This is due to two factors, the presence of proactive inhibition generated by previously presented training tasks and of retroactive inhibition produced by subsequently presented tasks. Both sources of interference can either serve to obscure retention differences due to the massive amounts of forgetting that can occur or to exaggerate any differences that may be present (cf. Underwood, 1957). Furthermore, learning one task might bias a subject's approach to the remaining tasks and hopelessly confound the data.

The only adequate solution to this problem is to have any one subject participate in only a single training task on Day 1. Though this may seem inefficient in terms of the number of subjects needed to complete an experiment and the amount of time spent running subjects, experience has shown us that it actually is economical in the long run, since it is the only way to collect usable data.

Summary

In summary, we believe that to demonstrate retention differences three design elements are critical:

1. The degree of learning needs to be equated properly with respect to the demands of the final retention task.

2. The degree of learning needs to be assessed shortly following learning by independent groups of subjects to assure that the groups are equivalent at the start of the retention interval.

3. Subjects must learn only a single task during the training session to eliminate proactive and retroactive inhibition and possible changes in a subject's learning strategy.

ACKNOWLEDGMENTS

Preparation of this paper was facilitated by research grant MH-10249 from the National Institute of Mental Health.

REFERENCES

Amster, H., Keppel, G., & Meyer, A. Learning and retention of letter pairs as a function of association strength. *American Journal of Psychology*, 1970, *83*, 22–39.

Bahrick, H. P. Retention curves: Facts or artifacts? *Psychological Bulletin*, 1964, *61*, 188–194.

Battig, W. F. Facilitation and interference. In E. A. Bilodeau (Ed.), *Acquisition of skill*. New York: Academic Press, 1966.

Battig, W. F. Paired-associate learning. In T. R. Dixon and D. L. Horton (Eds.), *Verbal behavior and general behavior theory*. Englewood Cliffs, N.J.: Prentice-Hall, 1968.

Bilodeau, E. A. Experimental interference with primary associates and their subsequent recovery with rest. *Journal of Experimental Psychology*, 1967, *73*, 328–332.

Bilodeau, I. McD., & Schlosberg, H. Similarity in stimulating conditions as a variable in retroactive inhibition. *Journal of Experimental Psychology*, 1951, *41*, 199–204.

Blake, M. J. F. Temperature and time of day. In W. P. Colquhoun (Ed.), *Biological rhythms and human performance*. London: Academic Press, 1971.

Briggs, G. E. Acquisition, extinction, and recovery functions in retroactive inhibition. *Journal of Experimental Psychology*, 1954, *47*, 285–293.

Colquhoun, W. P. (Ed.). *Biological rhythms and human performance*. London: Academic Press, 1971.

Craik, F. I. M., & Lockhart, R. S. Levels of processing: A framework for memory research. *Journal of Verbal Learning and Verbal Behavior*, 1972, *11*, 671–684.

Godden, D. R., & Baddeley, A. D. Context-dependent memory in two natural environments: On land and underwater. *British Journal of Psychology*, 1975, *66*, 325–331.

Greeno, J. G., James, C. T., & DaPolito, F. J. A cognitive interpretation of negative transfer and forgetting of paired associates. *Journal of Verbal Learning and Verbal Behavior*, 1971, *10*, 331–345.

Greenspoon, J., & Ranyard, R. Stimulus conditions and retroactive inhibition. *Journal of Experimental Psychology*, 1957, *53*, 55–59.

Hasher, L., Griffin, M., & Johnson, M. K. More on interpretive factors in forgetting. *Memory & Cognition*, 1977, *5*, 41–45.

Hasher, L., & Johnson, M. K. Interpretive factors in forgetting. *Journal of Experimental Psychology: Human Learning and Memory*, 1975, *1*, 567–575.

Holloway, F. A., & Wansley, R. A. Multiphasic retention deficits at periodic intervals after passive avoidance learning. *Science*, 1973, *180*, 208–210.

Hyde, T. S., & Jenkins, J. J. Recall for words as a function of semantic, graphic, and syntactic orienting tasks. *Journal of Verbal Learning and Verbal Behavior*, 1973, *12*, 471–480.

Joinson, P. A., & Runquist, W. N. Effects of intralist stimulus similarity and degree of learning on forgetting. *Journal of Verbal Learning and Verbal Behavior*, 1968, *7*, 554–559.

Keppel, G. Facilitation in short- and long-term retention of paired associates following distributed practice in learning. *Journal of Verbal Learning and Verbal Behavior*, 1964, *3*, 91–111.

Keppel, G. A reconsideration of the extinction–recovery theory. *Journal of Verbal Learning and Verbal Behavior*, 1967, *6*, 476–486.

Keppel, G. Retroactive and proactive inhibition. In T. R. Dixon & D. L. Horton (Eds.), *Verbal behavior and general behavior theory*. Englewood Cliffs, N.J.: Prentice-Hall, 1968.

Keppel, G. Forgetting. In C. P. Duncan, L. Sechrest, & A. W. Melton (Eds.), *Human memory: Festschrift for Benton J. Underwood.* New York: Appleton-Century-Crofts, 1972.

Keppel, G., Postman, L., & Zavortink, B. Studies of learning to learn: VIII. The influence of massive amounts of training upon the learning and retention of paired-associate lists. *Journal of Verbal Learning and Verbal Behavior*, 1968, *7*, 790–796.

Maltzman, I., Simon, S., Raskin, D., & Licht, L. Experimental studies in the training of originality. *Psychological Monographs*, 1960, *74*, (6, Whole No. 493).

Martin, E. Stimulus meaningfulness and paired-associate transfer: An encoding variability hypothesis. *Psychological Review*, 1968, *75*, 421–441.

Montague, W. E., Adams, J. A., & Kiess, H. O. Forgetting and natural language mediation. *Journal of Experimental Psychology*, 1966, *72*, 829–833.

Overton, D. A. Experimental methods for the study of state-dependent learning. *Federation Proceedings*, 1974, *33*, 1800–1813.

Paivio, A. *Imagery and verbal processes.* New York: Holt, Rinehart & Winston, 1971.

Peterson, R. C. Retrieval failures in alcohol state-dependent learning. Unpublished manuscript, 1976.

Posner, M. I. Psychobiology of attention. In M. S. Gazzaniga & C. Blakemore (Eds.) *Handbook of psychobiology*. New York: Academic Press, 1975.

Postman, L., Fraser, J., & Burns, S. Unit-sequence facilitation in recall. *Journal of Verbal Learning and Verbal Behavior*, 1968, *7*, 217–224.

Postman, L., & Keppel, G. Conditions of cumulative proactive inhibition. *Journal of Experimental Psychology: General*, in press.

Postman, L., & Stark, K. Role of response availability in transfer and interference. *Journal of Experimental Psychology*, 1969, *79*, 168–177.

Rand, G., & Wapner, S. Postural status as a factor in memory. *Journal of Verbal Learning and Verbal Behavior*, 1967, *6*, 268–271.

Rock, I. The role of repetition in associative learning. *American Journal of Psychology*, 1957, *70*, 186–193.

Shuell, T. J., & Keppel, G. Learning ability and retention. *Journal of Educational Psychology*, 1970, *61*, 59–65.

Strand, B. Z. Change of context and retroactive inhibition. *Journal of Verbal Learning and Verbal Behavior*, 1970, *9*, 202–206.

Tulving, E. Intratrial and intertrial retention: Notes towards a theory of free recall verbal learning. *Psychological Review*, 1964, *71*, 219–237.

Tulving, E., & Arbuckle, T. Y. Sources of intratrial interference in immediate recall of paired associates. *Journal of Verbal Learning and Verbal Behavior*, 1963, *1*, 321–334.

Tulving, E., & Osler, S. Effectiveness of retrieval cues in memory for words. *Journal of Experimental Psychology*, 1968, *77*, 593–601.

Turnage, T. W. Pre-experimental associative probability as a determinant of retention. *Journal of Verbal Learning and Verbal Behavior*, 1963, *2*, 352–360.

Underwood, B. J. Speed of learning and amount retained: A consideration of methodology. *Psychological Bulletin*, 1954, *51*, 276–282.

Underwood, B. J. Interference and forgetting. *Psychological Review*, 1957, *64*, 49–60.

Underwood, B. J. Degree of learning and the measurement of forgetting. *Journal of Verbal Learning and Verbal Behavior*, 1964, *3*, 112–129.

Underwood, B. J. Attributes of memory. *Psychological Review*, 1969, *76*, 559–573.

Underwood, B. J., & Keppel, G. Retention as a function of degree of learning and letter-sequence interference. *Psychological Monographs*, 1963, *77*, No. 4.

Underwood, B. J., Keppel, G., & Schulz, R. W. Studies of distributed practice: XXII. Some conditions which enhance retention. *Journal of Experimental Psychology*, 1962, *64*, 355–363.

Underwood, B. J., & Postman, L. Extraexperimental sources of interference in forgetting. *Psychological Review*, 1960, *67*, 73–95.

Underwood, B. J., Rehula, R., & Keppel, G. Item-selection in paired-associate learning. *American Journal of Psychology*, 1962, *75*, 353–371.

Underwood, B. J., & Schulz, R. W. Studies of distributed practice: XX. Sources of interference associated with differences in learning and retention. *Journal of Experimental Psychology*, 1961, *61*, 228–235.

Weingartner, H., & Murphy, D. State-dependent recall in manic depressive disorders. *Proceedings of the 82nd Annual Convention of the American Psychological Association*, 1974.

Part III

MEMORY AND ALCOHOL INTOXICATION

7

Acute Effects of Alcohol on Storage and Retrieval

Isabel M. Birnbaum

University of California at Irvine

Elizabeth S. Parker

National Institute on Alcohol Abuse and Alcoholism

As proceedings of the conference illustrate, a consistent property of alcohol is its capacity to alter memory processes. During acute intoxication, significant decrements occur in the ability to learn and recall new information (Jones & Jones, this volume; Parker, Alkana, Birnbaum, Hartley, & Noble, 1974; Ryback, 1971). Undoubtedly, the most severe instance of acute alcohol-related memory loss is the alcoholic blackout (Goodwin, this volume); however, even nonalcoholic subjects after ingesting relatively modest amounts of alcohol show decrements on a variety of memory tasks. In view of the reliable impairment of memory that is produced by alcohol, it seems particularly important to explore more fully the processes responsible for the impairment. Our current research is directed at determining whether separate stages of memory are differentially susceptible to acute doses of alcohol. This approach provides a foundation for exploring specific cognitive changes that occur under alcohol intoxication.

Our investigations have focused on distinguishing between the effects of alcohol on the phases of memory known as storage and retrieval. There are several lines of evidence that demand a distinction between the processes of storage of new information and subsequent retrieval of that information (Melton, 1963; Tulving, 1968). Items that have been stored in memory and are *potentially* available for recall are not necessarily retrievable. For example, after subjects have recalled all they can remember from a previously learned list of words, unrecalled items are suddenly recalled if the subject is provided with specific cues such as the names of categories to which items on the list belong.

Appropriate controls show that augmented recall after cuing is not simply the result of additional time for searching of memory or guessing; the cues can bring seemingly "unrecallable" material to the subject's consciousness (Allen, 1969; Tulving & Pearlstone, 1966; Tulving & Psotka, 1971). Another illustration of the storage–retrieval distinction is the "tip of the tongue" phenomenon, wherein information "escapes" one's memory for a period of time but seems to be very close to consciousness. Subjects who are experiencing a "tip of the tongue" state are often confident that they know the specific information in question and indeed are able to recognize it correctly at a later time (Blake, 1973; Brown & McNeill, 1966; Hart, 1967). In the more formal paired-associate learning situation, Nelson (1971) found that pairs that cannot be recalled after a two-week interval are relearned significantly more rapidly than are new pairs that have never been studied before. Again there was a utilizable "trace" of the original information even when the information could not be retrieved. In summary, the evidence from a wide range of studies points to the importance of distinguishing between different sources of decrements in memory. Has the information been adequately stored at the outset? Has there been a subsequent change in the characteristics of the stored information? Is the stored information retrievable? Conclusions about memory loss may depend upon whether storage or retrieval of the material is assessed and upon the techniques used for assessment.

Although the logical basis for our framework is straightforward, there are unresolved theoretical and methodological issues. How can storage be assessed without tapping retrieval processes, and vice versa? How sound is the rationale behind the methods that have been proposed to separate storage and retrieval? Each method relies on a number of assumptions. There is far from a clear-cut answer to the question, "Does alcohol affect storage, or retrieval, or both?" In this research effort as in others, ". . . as soon as one begins to consider how the question can be answered empirically, one is faced with an apparently endless sequence of restrictions and qualifications. . . . The end result of a research effort is rarely a clear answer to the original question; it is much more often a realization that the question can only be answered within the framework of an adequate theory [Estes, 1975, p. 123]." In exploring possible answers to the questions that we posed, we obtained some interesting and provocative results.

When a subject is presented with to-be-learned material and is later able to remember that material, we assume that a trace must have been formed (a storage process) and that information from the trace was searched for and found (a retrieval process). Within this framework, a substantial portion of research on alcohol-induced memory deficits does not permit an assessment of the relative contribution of alcohol's effects on storage and retrieval. Many of the tasks that were employed (e.g., free recall, paired-associate and serial learning, sentence memory) required both the acquisition of new information and retrieval of that information at the time of the test (Goodwin, Powell, Bremer, Hoine, & Stern,

1969; Jones, 1973; Parker et al., 1974; Storm & Caird, 1967; Tarter, 1970; Weingartner & Faillace, 1971).

STORAGE PROCESSES

Our initial work began with a search for tasks that either minimize the difficulty of retrieval or eliminate the necessity for retrieval. Of course, this implies that we know when retrieval is required and when it is hard or easy, but we do not. We made certain assumptions, and those assumptions must be evaluated as we proceed.

It has been widely held that accurate performance on a recognition test does not involve retrieval, that the subject simply matches the test item with his memorial representation of the items that were on the list. But is this memorial representation automatically there, or does the subject have to retrieve it before he can perform the matching task? Tulving and Thomson (1971) are the most persuasive advocates of the position that recognition memory requires retrieval; most theorists take the opposite position (see Tulving & Thomson, 1971, for a review). We assume that recognition memory does not require a search for the original information or, alternatively, that the search is very easy. Accordingly, an alcohol-induced impairment of recognition memory would be indicative of a deficit in storage processes. Two previous studies have found such impairments (Ryback, Weinert, & Fozard, 1970; Wickelgren, 1975), suggesting that the storage phase of memory is disrupted by alcohol intoxication.

Our first study expanded this line of research by using both a recognition task and a paired-associate task that was designed to minimize the difficulty of retrieval (Parker, Birnbaum, & Noble, 1976). A pilot study had shown that the 12 months of the year were readily recalled even under the highest dose to be used. We constructed paired-associate lists with the months of the year as responses, and subjects learned 12 consonant-month pairs after ingesting either a placebo drink, a medium dose, or a high dose of alcohol.[1] Registration was ensured on study trials by having the subjects read the pairs aloud, and the test trials were self-paced. Since the months were readily available, a failure to respond correctly on the test trials would not be attributable to impairment of retrieval of the response terms. Thus, the subject's task on a test trial was essentially the same as a matching task. After reaching a criterion of 100% correct or after 30 minutes had elapsed, subjects moved on to the next task, which was picture recognition.[2] Forty colored photographs of outdoor scenes

---

[1] The medium dose was .5 milliliters of alcohol per kilogram of body weight (ml/kg), and the high does was 1.0 ml/kg. For a 150-lb. subject, the high dose was approximately 5 $\frac{1}{2}$ oz. of 80-proof vodka mixed with an equal volume of masking solution.

[2] We thank Colin M. MacLeod for preparing materials and procedures for the task.

were shown at a 4-second rate. Subjects had been instructed to pay close attention to the details, because they would later be tested for recognition of the pictures. A two-alternative, forced-choice recognition test was given on a randomly selected 20 of the 40 target photographs. The distractors were highly similar scenes that differed only slightly from the targets. Given our assumptions regarding the minimal need for retrieval on these two tasks, alcohol-induced impairments of performance would be attributed to deficiencies in the process of storage. The strongest evidence for impairment of storage by alcohol would be the occurrence of dose-dependent deficits on both tasks. An alternative explanation based on motivational differences will also be considered.

On the paired-associate task, the learning curves for placebo and medium-dose subjects were almost identical, whereas high-dose subjects were significantly lower on trial 1 ($p < .01$) and remained consistently below the other two groups on subsequent trials. Different measures, for example, number correct per trial and trials to successive criteria, showed the same thing: only the high dose of alcohol impaired the acquisition of new associations on the paired-associate task. For picture recognition the story was a little different. There was a dose-dependent decrement in accuracy of recognition ($p < .05$). The mean number of correct responses was 16.4, 15.4, and 14.4 in the placebo, medium-, and high-dose groups, respectively.

One of the time-honored explanations of alcohol's detrimental effects on learning is that alcohol decreases motivation to perform well. We assessed motivational effects indirectly by measuring latency in the paired-associate task. We assumed that if a subject was uncertain about the accuracy of his response and he was motivated to respond correctly, he would take some time to think over his response. This assumption was supported by the finding that the median latency of responding was greater for incorrect responses (9 seconds) than correct responses (4 seconds), $p < .001$. Under the high dose of alcohol, if subjects were just responding to "get on with it" rather than making an effort to be correct, there should have been a smaller difference between the latency of correct and incorrect responses than in the other groups. The interaction of Dose X Correct vs. Incorrect, however, was far from significant, $F < 1.00$. There was thus little support for the assumption that subjects under the high dose of alcohol were not as well motivated as were subjects in the other two groups.

The results support the notion that the acquisition or storage of new information is impeded when subjects are intoxicated. The fact that the medium dose of alcohol impaired picture recognition but did not affect paired-associate learning suggests that alcohol-induced loss may be related to the storage demands of the task. Successful performance on the picture recognition task may require the storage of many details in the photographs of outdoor scenes. Intuitively, the paired-associate task appears to make smaller demands on storage processes. The reasons for storage deficits during intoxication remain to be investigated. It is interesting to note that studies of alcoholic Korsakoff patients also point to storage deficits as the source of impairment (Cermak & Butters, 1973).

Future research on processes involved in the storage of new information will provide new leads for an understanding of alcohol-induced deficits in memory. For example, alcohol may influence the depth of processing of new information (Craik & Lockhart, 1972; Craik, this volume), the efficiency of mediators that are formed during acquisition (Hasher & Johnson, 1975), the success of the selective filtering process (Keppel & Zubrzycki, this volume), or the subsequent consolidation of the trace (Landauer, this volume; McGaugh & Herz, 1972). The results, so far, point to the potential value of a fine-grained analysis of alcohol's influence on the storage phase of memory.

RETRIEVAL PROCESSES

In an effort to measure the effects of alcohol on the retrieval of information, we have investigated free-recall learning in sober and intoxicated subjects. Free recall is a useful tool for this analysis because it provides a number of different indices of retrieval deficits. Examination of the influence of alcohol on different measures of retrieval will give a more complete picture than would an analysis of any single measure.

As mentioned earlier, when cued recall is higher than noncued recall it is assumed that retrieval failure was responsible, in part, for the nonrecall of list items. Tulving and Pearlstone (1966) distinguish between *unavailability* of list items (storage deficits) and *inaccessibility* of list items (retrieval deficits). An index of the degree of retrieval deficit is provided by the difference between cued and noncued recall. Another approach was used by Tulving and Psotka (1971) in their analysis of the free recall of categorized lists of words in a retroactive inhibition paradigm. Total recall was expressed ". . . as a product of two independent measures, category recall and words-within-categories recall . . . [p. 2]." The results of their study as well as others cited by them suggest that impairments of category recall reflect inaccessibility of higher-order units rather than deficiencies in storage. Consistent with this view is the fact that the accessibility of higher-order units can be changed without affecting the average number of words recalled within these units.

We took two different paths in assessing the influence of alcohol on the process of retrieval. In the first study (Birnbaum, Parker, Hartley, & Noble, in preparation), 48 subjects learned and recalled a categorized free-recall list after ingesting either a placebo drink or an alcoholic beverage (1.0 ml/kg). The list contained 10 categories of 6 words per category and was presented in blocked order. After three study-test trials, subjects were given a fourth test trial on which they were cued with the category names. On the first three test trials, intoxicated subjects recalled fewer words, fewer words per category, and fewer categories than did sober subjects ($ps < .01$). If the recall of words within categories reflects storage, then the results are consistent with our previous conclusion that alcohol impairs the storage of new information. If the recall of categories reflects retrieval, then the observed deficits indicate that intoxicated subjects are also less well able to retrieve higher-order units. Results on the subsequent cued test trial indicate that there were retrieval deficits: when provided with category names, intoxicated subjects benefited significantly more than did sober subjects in total number of words recalled, and this was completely attributable to an increase in the number of categories recalled ($ps <$ .01). The results for the last trial of free recall and the subsequent tests of cued recall are shown in Table 1. The significant increase in words per category recalled ($p < .01$) was almost identical for both groups ($F < 1.00$) and was probably due to the longer period of time given on the cued trial. In summary, when they were given assistance in retrieval of higher-order units, intoxicated subjects showed a sharp increase in recall whereas sober subjects showed less improvement. One problem in interpreting these results is that sober subjects were close to ceiling in category recall, so there was more room for improvement in recall of higher-order units for intoxicated than for sober subjects. In spite of this problem, it does appear that sober subjects were better able to "empty the contents" of storage than were the intoxicated subjects on the preceding noncued test trial. It will be of interest to determine whether sober subjects are also better able to "empty the contents" of storage on the first and second test trials when they are not so close to ceiling.

The results of the study implicate deficits in retrieval as part of the memory impairment produced by alcohol intoxication. To test this implication more directly, we equated the storage of new material by having 48 subjects learn free-recall and paired-associate lists while they were sober in the first of two sessions (Birnbaum et al., in preparation). One week later, subjects were tested for recall of the lists while they were either sober or intoxicated (1.0 ml/kg). The tests of recall required retrieval, so if sober subjects were better able to "empty the contents" of storage, then their recall of the lists would be superior to that of intoxicated subjects. Next, a second test of recall was given in which the difficulty of retrieval was minimized (cued recall and matching). On the second test, any difference between sober and intoxicated subjects should be substantially reduced, since the retrieval requirements were minimized.

TABLE 1
Performance Measures in Free and Cued Recall

Condition		Number of words recalled	Number of categories recalled	Number of words per category
Sober	Free recall[a]	42.4	9.5	4.45
	Cued recall	46.5	10.0	4.65
Intoxicated	Free recall[a]	29.5	8.3	3.55
	Cued recall	37.2	9.9	3.74

[a]Trial 3 of Free Recall

In the first session the categorized free-recall list was presented for four study-test trials, and a paired-associate list (nine consonant—adjective pairs) was learned to a criterion of one perfect recitation. The free-recall list was presented auditorily by tape recorder, the paired-associate list was presented visually on slides, and the lists were learned in different rooms to increase differentiation between the tasks. As would be expected, since all subjects were sober, there were no significant differences between to-be-sober and to-be-intoxicated subjects on various measures of learning the lists in the first session (e.g., number correct in free recall and trials to criterion in paired-associate learning).

In the second session one week later, after receiving either a placebo drink or an alcoholic beverage, subjects were tested as follows: first a test of free recall of the categorized list was administered and was followed by either a cued or a noncued test of recall of the list. Then, recall of the paired-associate list was tested by presenting each consonant alone and asking for recall of the word that had been paired with it. The test was self-paced. After recall of the nine pairs had been tested, all subjects received a list of the nine adjectives and a second recall test was given. The subject had to indicate which of the nine adjectives had been paired with each consonant. In light of the implications of the previous study, the results were surprising to us. On the tests of recall that required retrieval, the sober and intoxicated subjects performed equally well. In free recall, a mean number of 26.0 and 24.5 words were recalled by the sober and intoxicated subjects, respectively, $F < 1.00$. On the first paired-associate test, the sober and intoxicated subjects recalled the same mean number of correct responses, 3.4. There was no significant difference between groups in the mean number of intrusions given in free recall ($F < 1.00$), discounting the possibility that intoxicated subjects inflated their scores by guessing more than did sober subjects. In summary, intoxicated and sober subjects were able to retrieve the same amount of previously learned material.

On the second tests of recall that minimized retrieval, sober and intoxicated subjects showed essentially the same amounts of improvement. For the free-recall list, sober and intoxicated subjects who were cued recalled a mean number of 39.1 and 38.0 words, respectively; whereas sober and intoxicated subjects who were not cued recalled a mean number of 30.8 and 28.8 words, respectively. The effect of cuing was significant, $F(1,44) = 9.1$, $p < .01$; and the effects of Dose and Dose $\times$ Cue were not significant, $Fs < 1.00$. Similarly, sober and intoxicated subjects showed essentially the same amount of improvement on the second paired-associate test, recalling a mean number of 6.5 and 6.8 correct pairs, respectively, $F < 1.00$.

The results of the first tests of recall in the second session, both of which required retrieval, indicate that an alcoholic beverage of 1.0 ml/kg (the same dose that had been used before) does not impair retrieval. These results suggest that the earlier observed differences between sober and intoxicated subjects during learning of the free-recall list (Table 1) may reflect solely a difference in storage processes. This conclusion is contradicted, however, by the fact that intoxicated subjects recalled fewer categories than did sober subjects during acquisition and more strongly contradicted by the fact that on the third free-recall test trial sober subjects recalled words from almost all *eventually recalled* categories whereas intoxicated subjects did not. These results suggest that on the noncued tests, intoxicated subjects had greater difficulty than did sober subjects in retrieving some of the stored information. Why then were intoxicated and sober subjects equally well able to retrieve previously learned information a week after it had been learned? Doesn't the first result predict retrieval deficits a week later? These results can be reconciled if it is assumed that sober subjects in the earlier study were able to "empty the contents" of storage on noncued test trials more thoroughly than intoxicated subjects only because the material was stored more strongly and not because they were superior in ability to retrieve. This possibility might be tested by bringing sober and intoxicated subjects to the same intermediate level of free recall and then providing them with category names as cues. If intoxicated subjects showed greater improvement under these circumstances, it could be more firmly concluded that they have a deficit in ability to retrieve learned information. If, on the other hand, sober and intoxicated subjects benefited equally when cues were provided at equivalent stages of learning, it would be likely that alcohol-induced deficits in free-recall learning do not reflect impairment of retrieval. Certainly the results of the recall tests given one week after original learning favor the conclusion that retrieval is not strongly influenced by alcohol intoxication.

SUMMARY

The results of these studies indicate that the storage of different types of information, verbal and visual, is impaired by acute doses of alcohol. In contrast, information previously learned in the sober state can be retrieved equally well under sober and intoxicated conditions. We offer the tentative conclusion that the strongest effects of acute alcohol intoxication on memory are to be found in the storage stage.

It is important not to overlook the fact that our studies were conducted with nonalcoholic subjects and the doses were well below the amounts that alcoholic individuals often consume. If large amounts of alcohol were ingested, a deterioration in retrieval processes might be observed. Even if this were the case, it would not weaken the conclusion that the storage phase of memory is more susceptible to disruption by alcohol than is the retrieval phase. The fact that chronic deficits also appear to be localized in the storage stage (Cermak & Butters, 1973) lends support to the hypothesis that there may be a continuum between memory deficits associated with acute intoxication and the chronic amnesia of Korsakoff's syndrome (Ryback, 1971).

Impairments in the ability to store new information imply a more permanent character to alcohol's effects on memory than would be the case if retrieval processes were disrupted. Alcohol-induced losses in retrieval would mean that during intoxication there is a reduction in the utilization of stored information, but upon return to sobriety memory functioning will recover. Deficits in storage, however, suggest that under the influence of alcohol weaker traces are being laid down. Thus, even upon return to sobriety, recall will be impaired for events experienced during intoxication. If these events are poorly stored, then their impact on the individual's behavior will be relatively weak. It has been suggested that therapy for alcoholic individuals might be more effective if it were conducted in the intoxicated state since this would counteract potential state-dependent losses in memory (Storm & Smart, 1965). However, our results indicate that these therapeutic efforts would be of little value unless they were conducted with the recognition that storage processes are impaired under the influence of alcohol.

The next phase of our research on alcohol and memory will address a number of important questions. Does alcohol alter the way new information is encoded? What techniques do intoxicated subjects use to learn new information? Are they using the same techniques as sober subjects, only less effectively, or are they using different techniques? Will alcohol-induced deficits in learning be reversed when intoxicated subjects are provided with techniques that sober subjects use spontaneously? Does alcohol impair the consolidation of memory traces? These are but a few of the avenues that research in this area may follow. There is little doubt that studies of alcohol and memory will continue to advance our understanding of alcohol's effects on behavior as well as to develop our knowledge about the workings of normal memory processes.

ACKNOWLEDGMENTS

The research described in this chapter was supported by research grant AA01468 from the National Institute on Alcohol Abuse and Alcoholism.

REFERENCES

Allen, M. M. Cueing and retrieval in free recall. *Journal of Experimental Psychology,* 1969, *81,* 29–35.

Birnbaum, I. M., Parker, E. S., Hartley, J. T., & Noble, E. P. Alcohol and memory: Retrieval processes. Manuscript in preparation.

Blake, M. Prediction of recognition when recall fails: Exploring the feeling-of-knowing phenomenon. *Journal of Verbal Learning and Verbal Behavior,* 1973, *12,* 311–319.

Brown, R., & McNeill, D. The "tip of the tongue" phenomenon. *Journal of Verbal Learning and Verbal Behavior,* 1966, *5,* 325–337.

Cermak, L., & Butters, N. Information processing deficits of alcoholic Korsakoff patients. *Quarterly Journal of Studies on Alcohol,* 1973, *34,* 1110–1132.

Craik, F. I. M., & Lockhart, R. S. Levels of processing: A framework for memory research. *Journal of Verbal Learning and Verbal Behavior,* 1972, *11,* 671–684.

Estes, W. K. The locus of inferential and perceptual processes in letter identification. *Journal of Experimental Psychology: General,* 1975, *104,* 122–145.

Goodwin, D. W., Powell, B., Bremer, D., Hoine, H., & Stern, J. Alcohol and recall: State-dependent effects in man. *Science,* 1969, *163,* 1358–1360.

Hart, J. T. Memory and the memory-monitoring process. *Journal of Verbal Learning and Verbal Behavior,* 1967, *6,* 685–691.

Hasher, L., & Johnson, M. K. Interpretive factors in forgetting. *Journal of Experimental Psychology: Human Learning and Memory,* 1975, *1,* 567–575.

Jones, B. M. Memory impairment on the ascending and descending limbs of the blood alcohol curve. *Journal of Abnormal Psychology,* 1973, *82,* 24–32.

McGaugh, J. L., & Herz, M. J. *Memory consolidation.* San Francisco: Albion Publishing Co., 1972.

Melton, A. W. Implications of short-term memory for a general theory of memory. *Journal of Verbal Learning and Verbal Behavior,* 1963, *2,* 1–21.

Nelson, T. O. Savings and forgetting from long-term memory. *Journal of Verbal Learning and Verbal Behavior,* 1971, *10,* 568–576.

Parker, E. S., Alkana, R. L., Birnbaum, I. M., Hartley, J. T., & Noble, E. P. Alcohol and the disruption of cognitive processes. *Archives of General Psychiatry,* 1974, *31,* 824–828.

Parker, E. S., Birnbaum, I. M., & Noble, E. P. Alcohol and memory: Storage and state dependency. *Journal of Verbal Learning and Verbal Behavior,* 1976, *15,* 691–702.

Ryback, R. S. The continuum and specificity of the effects of alcohol on memory: A review. *Quarterly Journal of Studies on Alcohol,* 1971, *32,* 995–1016.

Ryback, R. S., Weinert, J., & Fozard, J. L. Disruption of short-term memory in man following consumption of ethanol. *Psychonomic Science,* 1970, *20,* 353–354.

Storm, T., & Caird, W. K. The effects of alcohol on serial verbal learning in chronic alcoholics. *Psychonomic Science,* 1967, *9,* 43–44.

Storm, T., & Smart, R. G. Dissociation: A possible explanation of some features of alcoholism and implications for treatment. *Quarterly Journal of Studies on Alcohol,* 1965, *26,* 111–115.

Tarter, R. E. Dissociate effects of ethyl alcohol. *Psychonomic Science,* 1970, *20,* 342–343.

Tulving, E. Theoretical issues in free recall. In T. R. Dixon & D. L. Horton (Eds.), *Verbal behavior and general behavior theory.* Englewood Cliffs, New Jersey: Prentice-Hall, 1968.

Tulving, E., & Pearlstone, Z. Availability versus accessibility of information in memory for words. *Journal of Verbal Learning and Verbal Behavior,* 1966, *5,* 381–391.

Tulving, E., & Psotka, J. Retroactive inhibition in free recall: Inaccessibility of information available in the memory store. *Journal of Experimental Psychology,* 1971, *87,* 1–8.

Tulving, E., & Thomson, D. M. Retrieval processes in recognition memory: Effects of associative context. *Journal of Experimental Psychology,* 1971, *87,* 116–124.

Weingartner, H., & Faillace, L. A. Alcohol and state-dependent learning in man. *Journal of Nervous and Mental Disease,* 1971, *153,* 395–406.

Wickelgren, W. Alcoholic intoxication and memory storage dynamics. *Memory & Cognition,* 1975, *3,* 385–389.

8

The "Intoxicated" Goldfish as a Model for Alcohol Effects on Memory in Humans

Ralph S. Ryback, M.D.

Intramural Research Division
NIAAA

Among the problems of patients presented at alcoholism clinics, the alcohol-induced "blackout" is often observed. Jellinek (1952) defined blackouts as memory lapses occurring after moderate drinking unaccompanied by signs of intoxication where the drinker "may carry on a reasonable conversation or go through quite elaborate activities without a trace of memory the next day [p. 678]." Jellinek found that blackouts after "medium" alcohol consumption were characteristic of the "prospective alcohol addict" and felt that, for the "great majority" of alcoholics, blackouts had prognostic significance in signaling the initial phase of addiction. Keller and Seeley (1958) defined the blackout as "amnesia for the events of any part of a drinking episode without loss of consciousness [p. 20]." – a definition applied in a study by Goodwin, Crane and Guze (1969), utilizing a structured interview with 100 hospitalized alcoholics. Ninety percent of their subjects who reported frequent blackouts attributed it to increased consumption of alcohol.

Although blackouts are often associated with alcoholism, the phenomenon is by no means limited to alcoholics. Roe found that 30% of 30 middle-aged social drinkers had experienced blackouts (Jellinek, 1946); and Goodwin, Crane, and Guze (1969) found that almost 40% of nonalcholic men had experienced a blackout at least once. The men reporting blackouts were generally *lighter* drinkers than were those without such a history. Typically, they had been drunk once or twice and on one or both of these occasions experienced memory loss. It may be, as Goodwin, Crane, and Guze (1969) suggest, that *early* blackouts predict *non*alcoholism rather than alcoholism. This may be true, because fewer blackouts are induced by a given level of alcohol consumption after development of "tolerance" by the alcoholic.

Although the blackout phenomenon is a common and important symptom of excessive drinking, only a few experimental studies of alcohol amnesia in humans are available. In alcoholics, Diethelm and Barr (1962a) and Heber and Kryspin— Exner (1966) gave enough alcohol, intravenously or by mouth, respectively, to raise the blood alcohol concentration (BAC) to between 0.15% and 0.2% within 30 minutes. They both found that 24 hours later, there was substantial amnesia for what had occurred during the period of intoxication that followed. Hutchison, Tuchtie, Gray, and Steinberg (1964) found similar results with several nonalcoholic subjects.

Interpretations of the blackout phenomenon vary. Diethelm and Barr (1962b) interpret such amnesia in psychodynamic terms, rather than as a disruption of neurophysiological or neurochemical mechanisms of information storage, suggesting such dynamics as: (1) escape from self; (2) reduction of tension, alertness, or motivation; and (3) expression of dissociated impulses (Washburne, 1958).

In addition to "blackouts," clinic patients often report what they call the "greyout" — a phenomenon that seems to occur after a period of moderately heavy drinking and that is characterized by an ability to recall what happened if companions describe some of the events. On several occasions they also recalled events that occurred while drinking when they became similarly intoxicated. This phenomenon will be discussed later in terms of our recent knowledge of state-dependent learning (Overton, 1966).

There are good reasons — both clinical and theoretical — for making a further analysis of "alcohol amnesia" effects in humans. First of all, we should regard memory deficits as characteristic symptoms of alcohol intoxication. Understanding alcohol's action upon memory provides general hints as to its pharmacological properties. Secondly, the short-term impairments induced by high blood-alcohol levels may be related to the etiology of chronic memory impairments, as seen in the Korsakoff syndrome. Third, the alcoholic's loss of memory for events occurring during drinking bouts may impose a barrier for psychotherapy. Further understanding of mechanisms of "dissociation" between alcohol and sober states might provide hints for the therapist — e.g., suggest the possibility of doing therapy while the patient is inebriated. Finally, we suggest that alcohol may prove the most convenient drug for experimental alteration of memory states in man. Now that a rich assortment of analytical memory tests are available to probe the factors that limit stages of encoding, storage, and retrieval of information, a judicious use of alcohol might assist those theorists who wish to experimentally fractionate the underlying components of memory.

EXPERIMENTAL APPROACHES TO MEMORY DISRUPTION

Although there is a large literature on neurological correlates of memory loss and neurophysiological correlates of memory formation, we take a conservative view of these data and do not believe that they support any particular hypothesis concerning "physical mechanisms" of memory formation. Our discussion of modifications of memory by alcohol is confined to "psychological" processes on the one hand and "neurochemical" hypotheses on the other (Shashoua, 1975). In this article, we shall consider evidence from humans and animals that alcohol may disrupt particular stages of memory formation without attempting to localize these critical events within the brain. For the present, we accept the popular distinctions between (1) sensory registration or "immediate" memory (IM), (2) "short-term" memory (STM), and (3) semipermanent or "long-term" memory (LTM). This tripartite model of memory stages is among the alternatives reviewed by Sheer (1970). In the first stage, information is held temporarily in a buffer storage until it is attended to and processed more fully. As Sperling (1960) and others have shown, such information may dissipate in a matter of seconds. Recent research further supports the concept of IM or sensory registration. Sakitt (1975) found that visual immediate memory (i.e., iconic memory) is primarily located in the retina at the level of the photoreceptors. It is our view that other peripheral receptors play a similar role. Moreover, a study by Moskowitz and Murray (1976) found that alcohol increased the time necessary to transfer information from the initial sensory information storage system into the STM system. Nevertheless, the tripartite hypothesis suggests the STM stage is more selective than IM and can accept only a limited amount of information at any one moment. However, verbal encoding or other cognitive strategies ("chunking" related bits of information) can increase the efficiency of the STM phase of storage. Therefore, allowing a subject to rehearse these encoding strategies or process the information at "different levels" (Craik, this volume) will strikingly improve later recall of information.

Although various workers report vastly different posttraining intervals wherein STM can be disrupted, (e.g., by electroconvulsive shock), there is general agreement that LTM can be disrupted by drug treatments many minutes after training (e.g., Agranoff & Klinger, 1964; Agranoff, 1967). Data obtained from training and retention tests with mice and goldfish support the notion that a labile STM process is gradually "fixed" into the LTM mode and that many minutes or even hours are required to complete the transition. From this point of view, alcohol might antagonize memory formation through any of the following effects:

1. Interference with the encoding of raw information from IM into "chunks" for STM storage.

2. Alteration of the rate of decay of STM once primary information has been entered.

3. Disruption of the fixation of short-term molecular changes into a stable, long-term representation.

4. Reduction of the accessibility of the once-formed engram to later "read-out."

Psychological hypotheses might concern: (1) arousal level required to sustain STM processes; (2) cognitive level required to effectively "chunk" information; or (3) use of strategies and available cues for later retrieval of stored information.

These alternatives are by no means a complete list of theoretically viable possibilities, but they do hint at the complexity of the experimental problem.

Can we approach clinical phenomena of alcohol amnesia in terms of the serial stage theory of memory formation? We are encouraged in this approach by noting the effects that "hippocampal-temporal" lesions may have in humans: normal IM processing and good cognitive capacity coexistent with striking loss of later recall (Milner, 1959). Is is possible that alcohol can wipe out STM or LTM storage without significantly depressing initial registration of information (IM)? One study approached this question by testing normal subjects with a picture—recognition task during moderate levels of alcohol intoxication (Ryback, Weinert, & Fozard, 1970). It was found that alcohol disrupted recognition for pictures presented minutes earlier but did not depress immediate memory capacities. Similar results were observed in intoxicated alcoholics (Ryback, 1970a) where alcohol appeared to specifically disrupt STM, leaving intact both IM and LTM for skills, information, and events that occurred prior to inebriation. The drinking session had no effect upon later LTM, except for those events that occurred during the session. Because the STM phase can be disrupted, it was not possible in these experiments to further test the possibility that transition from STM to LTM might also be disrupted by alcohol as occurs in animals treated with antimetabolic drugs. Our experimental demonstration agrees well with common anecdotal reports of alcoholics — e.g., a patient who becomes severely intoxicated in a bar, pays his bill, drives home, yet wakes up the next day with no memory of these events. Since, in many cases, neither reintoxication nor cuing the subject aids recall, we presume that the critical information was never effectively entered into LTM.

The findings of a deficit in STM processing in alcoholics and nonalcoholics resulted in a hypothesis (Ryback, 1971) of a "continuum" in STM disruption from cocktail party memory deficits to alcohol amnesia to the Wernicke—Korsakoff memory impairment. Findings of a recent controlled study (Cermak & Ryback, 1976) appear to support this idea. Patients with a history of chronic alcoholism given a STM test 24 hours after their admission presented Korsakoff-like memory impairments and a STM deficit similar to that found in subjects experiencing alcohol amnesia, particularly if they were more than 50 years of age. However, their STM slowly improved over a period of several weeks until they were not distinguishable from normal controls. Other published data (Ilchysin & Ryback, 1976) further support the idea of a "continuum" in that alcoholic patients with a frequent history of blackouts had significant impairments in their STM after 3 weeks of sobriety, whereas those with no history of blackout showed either no signs or few signs of deficit.

Neverthelsss, there is controversy within the literature on amnesia as to whether Korsakoff patients have an intact or impaired STM. Warrington and Weiskrantz (1973) have presented evidence to suggest that amnesia is a deficit in LTM with STM essentially normal, but Cermak and Butters (1972), Cermak, Butters, and Gerrein (1973), and Butters and Cermak (1975) have argued that Warrington is testing a subject population different from theirs. They have provided examples of patients whose main deficits are a gross impairment in STM. A similar controversy has arisen around the effects of alcohol on STM in humans. Goodwin, Othmer, Halikas, and Freemon (1970), Tamerin, Weiner, Poppen, Steinglass, and Mendelson (1971) and Ryback (1970a) all found impairment in STM in intoxicated alcoholics; whereas Mello (1973) did not. Carpenter and Ross (1965), Nash (1962), and Ryback et al. (1970) have demonstrated disruption of visual STM in nonalcoholics with relatively low doses of alcohol. It is likely that the latter discrepant findings are in part related to a number of variables, including the definitions of STM used (Shuttleworth & Morris, 1966; McNamee, Mello, & Mendelson, 1968; Tamerin et al., 1971), the types of subjects used, the amounts of absolute alcohol consumed in a given time, and the types of STM tests (e.g., verbal or nonverbal). Accordingly, an experimental model that might better define some of these variables and test nonverbal "STM" and "LTM" would be helpful.

THE FISH AS A MODEL SYSTEM

Within the last decade several laboratories have utilized the goldfish for analytical studies of memory formation in relationship to RNA and protein synthesis theories of memory storage (Agranoff, 1967; Shashoua, 1968, 1970). Utilizing aftershock avoidance as a technique, Riege and Cherkin (1971) have provided data compatible with the two-store theory of memory formation. (Our choice of the fish as a model system for alcohol-related studies is ironic, in that the term "fish" has long been used as a euphemism for the human inebriate, "stewed to the gills" being a familiar expression.) Preliminary studies were carried out on memory phenomena in intoxicated goldfish (Ryback, 1969a) and on aggressive enhancement by alcohol in the Siamese Fighting Fish (Raynes, Ryback, & Ingle, 1968). Since amnesia and hyperaggressive behaviors (Shupe, 1954) are characteristic of both fish and human under appropriate alcohol levels, there were explicit advantages in the use of fish for such research (e.g., Ryback, 1970b).

The chief advantage in the use of a fish model was its comparative simplicity in brain structure and its stereotyped behavior. Although fish probably store much less information during their lives than do mammals, a review of Bitterman (1969) indicates that they learn quickly and remember well a variety of tasks that are within their behavioral repertoire. It is important to emphasize that goldfish (and other species) can acquire simple visual discriminations (Savage & Swingland, 1969; Nolte, 1933), maze tasks (Ingle, 1965b), and classical conditioning (Bernstein, 1961; Overmier & Savage, 1974) in absence of the entire telencephalon. A similar operation in the mammal would leave the animal in a nearly vegetative state. It is possible in a fish, therefore, to dissociate memory phenomena from structures such as the neocortex (which they do not have) or hippocampal region, which is easily removed by ablation. The logistical problems of sampling neural subsystems in memory research should be simplified proportionately by restricting one's search to diencephalic and mesencephalic regions.

Structural and functional homologies are more obvious between fish and mammal at these diencephalic and mesencephalic levels. For example, the optic tectum subserves some homologous visuomotor functions from fish to primate (Ingle, 1973a). Stimulation of hypothalamus via implanted electrodes can elicit feeding or aggressive behaviors in teleost fish (Demski & Knigge, 1971) as well as in various mammals and birds. Hypothalamic lesions can lead to "visual neglect" in both goldfish (Regestein, 1968) and rats (Marshall, Turner, & Teitelbaum, 1971). We should not forget that studies of single-unit responses during conditioning of rats (Olds, Disterhoft, & Segal, 1972) found "learning foci" in thalamus, hypothalamus, and tegmentum in addition to telencephalon. A subcortical substrate for memory storage absolutely required for fish seems plausible for mammals as well, although the situation is certainly more complex in more highly differentiated mammalian brains. Thus, though we chose fish largely for relative simplicity of memory function, there is a good chance that some memory mechanisms in fish are anatomically homologous to those in mammals. Thus, any similarities in effects of alcohol on memory phenomena between fish and humans will at least suggest the possibility that alcohol can disrupt subcortical memory mechanisms in humans (Table 1).

A major technical advantage of fish is their ability to come into equilibrium with the surrounding solution of ethanol. The goldfish BAC reaches about 85% of the alcohol concentration in the surrounding aqueous environment (Ryback, Percarpio, & Vitale, 1969), whereas the convict cichlid shows a somewhat lower BAC at equilibrium (Peeke, Ellman, & Herz, 1973). Since fish can indefinitely remain at this steady-state level where BAC is neither rising nor falling during training, they prove ideal for learning studies and for tolerance studies where BAC cannot be altered by adaptation via the liver's capacity to metabolize ethanol.

TABLE 1

Neuropathology in Humans Resulting from Disease or Surgery that have Demonstrable Memory Defects, Compared to the Anatomical Homologues in the Goldfish (Ebbesson, 1972; Bernstein, 1970; Schnitzlein, 1968; Schulman, 1964; Adams, 1969; Pribram, 1969).

Areas lesioned in humans	Anatomical homologues in the goldfish
1. Bilateral lesions of the frontal association cortex.	1. No cortex present.
2. Lesions in the medial diencephalon, especially the medial dorsal thalamic nuclei.	2. Reticular core to medial thalamus.
3. Lesions of the medial parts of the temporal lobes, particularly the hippocampal and perihippocampal convolutions, the amygdala, and the fornices.	3. No temporal lobes present, but rudimentary "hippocampal and perihippocampal" and "amygdaloid region" are present.
4. Lesions of the medial and inferior parts of one or both temporal lobes.	4. No temporal lobe present.

Studies of Memory Deficits in the Intoxicated Goldfish

First, an attempt was made to simulate the blackout effect commonly experienced in human patients. Goldfish were trained (Ryback, 1969a) in a positional discrimination (i.e., to turn either left or right) in a simple Y-maze (Ingle, 1965a), by placing an invisible glass barrier just beyond the incorrect turn. Fish would normally learn this task within 30 trials to a criterion of 18/20 correct turns; and when trained at a moderate alcohol level (400 mg% — which would be severe for man), they would actually do somewhat better than this (Table 2). Immediately following training, one group of subjects was placed within a high alcohol solution (700 mg%) for 1 hour, which rapidly brought the BAC up to a depressive level. The fish, in fact, looked sluggish and many turned over on their sides within the hour.

Control fish trained at 400 mg% showed excellent memory for the learned habit 3 days later, even though tested in the same alcohol solution. However, those fish that were immediately blacked out by the high alcohol level did not retain their habit when tested 3 days later in the 400 mg% solution. A third group that was trained at 400 mg% returned to normal water and then blacked out 24 hours after the training test, but did show good retention on Day 3. From these data we conclude that memory formation must be disrupted within 1 hour after learning in order to prevent later retention. Furthermore, the effect of immediate blackout must be retroactive on consolidation of learning rather than proactive upon test performance.

Unfortunately, such variables as "difficulty," the training retention interval, and dose-dependent curves of learning and memory with alcohol have not been

TABLE 2

Trials to Criterion in Y-maze. Fish were trained in either 650 mg.% or
400 mg.% ethanol (Groups 1 and 2) after being in the same solution for 2
hours (No. 1–10, 17–26) or 6 hours (No. 11–16, 27–32), respectively.
Group 3 was trained in water. These results are from pooling together and
reanalyzing similarly treated fish in a previous experiment (Ryback, 1969b).

| | Group 1 | | Group 2 | | Group 3 |
| | Alcohol (2 & 6 hrs. | | Alcohol (2 & 6 hrs. | | |
No.	650 mg.%)	No.	400 mg.%)	No.	Water
1	59	17	10	33	28
2	100	18	10	34	30
3	6	19	8	35	81
4	5	20	25	36	25
5	57	21	6	37	46
6	96	22	27	38	8
7	60	23	13	39	14
8	144	24	9	40	21
9	8	25	10	41	35
10	68	26	14	42	22
11	40	27	4	43	9
12	41	28	30	44	15
13	26	29	6	45	22
14	21	30	8	46	34
15	27	31	9	47	21
16	44	32	21	48	45
Mean score:	50.1[a]		13[b]		28.5

[a]P < .025 in the direction predicted (t-test, Group 1 compared to Group 3).
[b]P < .001 in the direction predicted (t-test, Group 2 compared to Group 3).

thoroughly studied in fish. Is it possible to have amnesia *without* initial depression or good retention *despite* initial depression? Is the important difference
in procedure the training–retention interval? Is it possible that a 24-hour test
does not reveal the memory deficit that can be found after 3 days? Although
this suggestion might seem a bit strained, such data are reported for posttraining
effects of puromycin treatment of goldfish (Agranoff, 1967): fish show significant retention of an avoidance test at 24 hours, but memory has decayed
entirely by the 72-hour test. Obviously, this unsatisfactory state of knowledge
can be remedied by variation of both alcohol dosage and time of retesting after
either training under alcohol or after high-alcohol blackouts. Can LTM be
disrupted without a substantial impairment of STM? This question deserves

careful attention, since a positive answer would imply that alcohol may affect the interface between STM and LTM as claimed for antimetabolic drugs and electroconvulsive shock (McGaugh, 1970). A study of effects of alcohol upon the more subtle measures of RNA and protein synthesis (Shashoua, 1975) would then seem to be indicated.

In seeking parallels between fish and humans, we should also consider the interesting condition, state-dependent learning, or the ability to remember a task initially learned in a drugged state only when the subject is similarly drugged during the retention test. Overton (1971) described a number of examples of state-dependent learning in rats, primarily in experiments with tranquilizers or with depressants such as barbiturates. Descriptions of a similar phenomenon are often given by members of Alcoholics Anonymous: the individual remembers what transpired during the drinking session only when re-intoxicated. Objective verification of this phenomenon in humans was given by Storm and Caird (1967) and by Goodwin, Powell, Bremer, Hoine, & Stern (1969b). Must we refer this type of selective memory loss to such psychodynamic explanations as "repression" of painful memories? If we could demonstrate state-dependent memory effects in animals under alcohol intoxication, we might be more inclined to view the human memory failure as resulting from an inevitable pharmacological blockade, rather than from an emotional barrier.

Using the Y-maze test for goldfish, memory does prove to be state dependent, as with rats and human subjects (Ryback, 1969c). Goldfish remembered their maze habit best either when trained and tested sober or when trained and tested during intoxication (600 mg%), but not when switched from one state to the other. At lower alcohol levels (400 mg%), the dissociation was unidirectional; memory failure occurred only when going from alcohol to the sober state, but was transferred well in the reverse direction. This asymmetry in dissociation has been found in human studies (Storm & Caird, 1967; Goodwin, Powell, Bremer, Hoine, & Stern, 1969b) and with rats (Crow, 1966; Overton, 1971) and sustains the generality of our fish data. State-dependent memory effects have been confirmed for goldfish by studies of Richardson (1972), using a spatial discrimination method, and by Scobie and Bliss (1974), using an avoidance conditioning method.

Thus far, our goldfish model has shown two major similarities to man: alcohol intoxication can induce either blackout with complete amnesia as a consequence or, during less severe insult, can result in state-dependent memory loss. A major unsolved question for human studies concerns the localization of alcohol-induced impairments to the STM or LTM phase of memory formation. Can the goldfish model be used to approach this question on a simpler level where cognitive strategies of STM encoding would not be involved?

The following "gedanken experiment" (Ryback, 1976) illustrates the potential leverage offered by our fish model. Goldfish were overtrained on a positional habit, such that LTM was firmly established. This was already achieved in a pilot test by training fish to escape a dark box by swimming out the right side of a two-door apparatus. When our fish were then forced to escape for 10 trials via the "wrong" door (by covering the preferred right side), they were at first confused but soon accepted the new rules. If after a 5-minute (STM) delay both doors were then uncovered, intoxicated fish tended to persist in choosing the left side. A pilot study suggested that if the same fish were removed from the tank and returned in 1 hour, they reverted to an 80% choice of the original (right) door. It would seem that the strength of STM favoring the left door decays relative to the strength of LTM favoring the right door, and eventually the fish is relieved of its confusion. The results suggest that alcohol intoxication temporarily facilitates the STM of the forced reversal information; or, as Landauer (this volume) might suggest, the intoxicated animal is fixed in his "memory map," unable to properly scan for past or "more distant" information and thus perseverates at that which he has just learned.

To further support this suggestion, research would necessitate the addition of various alcohol concentrations and groups with varying time-delay intervals after the 10 conflictual trials so that a gradient from STM to LTM alcohol effects could be delineated. This memory model could also be used to study the effect of chronic alcohol exposure and the onset of symptoms in young and older goldfish as well as their resolution or improvement following cessation of alcohol exposure. This is clinically relevant, as Cermak and Ryback (1976) found that older alcoholics (age range 52–68) were particularly prone to experience an alcohol-induced STM deficit from which they slowly recovered over a 4-week interval of complete sobriety. Similarly, Illchysin and Ryback (1976) found that a history of blackouts was predictive of memory deficits in only the older age group (50–59).

ALCOHOL ENHANCEMENT OF LEARNING

In 1892, Kraepelin reported that impairment of human performance by large doses of alcohol was frequently preceded by improved performance on certain tasks. This paradoxical enhancement effect lasted longer after smaller alcohol doses, but was quite transient at higher levels. Such bimodal effects have been confirmed for human subjects (Carpenter, Moore, Snyder, & Lisansky, 1961) and extended to rats, using a conditioned avoidance test of learning (Crow, 1966; Holloway, 1972). An earlier maze study showed that the enhancement effect could be generalized to the goldfish as well (Ryback, 1969b). As Table 2 shows, goldfish in 400 mg% alcohol learned the left–vs–right discrimination significantly faster than did their sober controls. The enhancement effect has also been found by others using smaller fish trained in an avoidance task and under still higher alcohol levels (Petty, Bryant, & Byrne, 1973; Bryant, Petty,

Warren, & Byrne, 1973; Scobie & Bliss, 1974). It should be mentioned that fish studies have not used more complicated learning paradigms. These simple tasks might be better performed, because the fish is more active or less "nervous" and not because he is operating at the peak of mental capacity.

Actually, Ingle (1965b) reported a similar enhancement of goldfish learning in the Y-maze following total ablation of the telencephalon. In this instance, data analysis showed that lesioned fish were slightly slower in reaching an early 9/10 learning criterion but then went on to attain the 18/20 criterion significantly faster than their controls. Because the control subjects often ruined their successful runs with two or more successive errors, it appeared that these fish showed a "compulsion" to change direction that the lesioned animals did not show. The fish without telencephalon may have been "superior" due to lack of strong competing behaviors – i.e., "simplifying" the fish's approach to his task allowed him to fully attend to the simple turning habit.

We suspect that alcohol may also simplify the goldfish's behavior and thus reduce error-making tendencies, just as it increases the frequency of an un-learned avoidance jumping response in the common frog, due, we believe, to reduction of a competing tendency – freezing when frightened (Ingle, 1973a). Such a mechanism is also suggested by other kinds of studies where alcohol appears to "disinhibit" unlearned behaviors. Examples include reduction stimuli as prey (Ingle, 1973b) and prolongation of postrotary nystagmus in both fish and frogs (Ingle, 1973c).

The popular image of the goldfish is that of the dime-store pet who measures perhaps only 2 inches long. However, goldfish grow to more than 12 inches long, and as they mature their behavior changes noticeably. A review of the literature suggests that juvenile goldfish are less sensitive to alcohol's depressive or in-hibitory effects than adult goldfish (Table 3). Instead of darting about ner-vously, the larger fish are more leisurely and deliberate in their movements. Perhaps related to this mature calmness, the larger fish have much higher brain concentrations of serotonin (Shashoua, personal communication, 1975). As diverse experimental data suggest that reduction of brain serotonin is associated

TABLE 3
The Relationship of Alcohol Dose to Size and Facilitation or Inhibition of Learned Behavior with the Supporting References.

Size (inches)	Facilitation	Inhibition
1½ to 2	745 & 1100 mg.% (Bryant, Petty, Warren, & Byrne, 1973; Petty, Bryant, & Byrne, 1973).	
3 to 4	628 & 856 mg.% (Savage & Swingland, 1969).	
5 to 6	400 mg.% (Table 2)	650 mg.% (Ryback, 1969b).

with arousal states (Ryback, 1973), we were interested in comparing alcohol effects on fish of various sizes in the following unpublished experiment.

Using a position discrimination task (Ryback, 1976), the subjects were 25 "common goldfish" 3 to 4 inches long (average weight 12.9 grams) and 25 "common goldfish" 6 inches long (average weight 28.4 grams) obtained from the Ozark Fisheries (Stoutland, Missouri) in mid-August and tested from 1 to 4 weeks after habituation to the laboratory. Four small (3- to 4-inch) and 4 large (6-inch) goldfish were lost during initial training through illness or accident, so that the remaining 42 fish were randomly divided into 3 groups (i.e., A, B, and C), each of 7 small and 7 large fish respectively (Table 4). The door used for original training was that opposite each subject's spontaneous preference. Training proceeded as follows: (1) a criterion of 9 out of 10 correct choices was used and subjects were allowed up to 30 trials; (2) the following day, fish in groups A and B were given up to 30 "reversal" trials in the opposite direction (i.e., a fish trained on "right door" was forced to choose the "left door" by covering the "trained" or right door with the "invisible" glass barrier). Subjects in Group A were placed in alcohol solutions of 600 mg% for 3 hours and then given the reversal trials in this same solution; subjects in Group B were given the reversal trials in water. All subjects in Group C received training only on the original task; they were placed in alcohol solutions of 700 mg% for 3 hours and were then trained in this same solution. We found (Table 4) that a dose of 600 or 700 mg% for three hours would strikingly depress a 6- inch long fish in original or reversal training but would have no noticeable effect on the learning abilities of 3- to 4-inch long subjects.

Could the resistance of smaller fish be related to their lower levels of brain serotonin? Goldfish 3 to 4 inches long have approximately one-half the total brain concentration as goldfish 6 inches long (Shashoua, personal communication, 1975). Further support for this possibility came from observations that goldfish could be protected against depression from alcohol during maze learning if they either were (a) injected with parachlorophenyllanine; or (b) stressed by swimming upside down (Ingle, unpublished data, 1975). Either treatment tends to deplete brain serotonin in goldfish (Shashoua, 1975, and unpublished data). We do not suggest that alcohol directly depresses behavior by acting on serotonin metabolism, but we want to reinforce the view that effects of alcohol on behavior can vary considerably depending upon the emotional or neurochemical state of the organism. Furthermore, the finding that a hyperaroused goldfish is not retarded by a normally depressive alcohol dose raises the prospect of a more definitive answer to earlier questions about alcohol amnesia — whether alcohol impairs short-term memory by reduction of arousal or by its effect on serotonin (Ryback, 1973); whether alcohol blocks the transition of STM to LTM or whether 700 mg% alcohol would impair 3-day memory in fish protected from initial learning deficits by stress or in very small fish who learn well at this level. If the arousal state had nothing directly to do with efficacy of permanent

TABLE 4

Scores to Criterion (9 out of 10 Correct) for 3 Groups (A, B, and C) of Small (3- to 4-inch) and Large (6-inch) Goldfish, Using a Position Discrimination Task.

	Original task	Reversal task	Original task	Reversal task
	Small		Large	
Group A	Water	Alcohol 600 mg.%	Water	Alcohol 600 mg.%
	7	8	21	30
	8	7	10	30
	12	5	13	6
	18	4	8	16
	9	5	17	30
	15	7	13	23
	11	6	10	30
Mean:	11.4	6	13.1	23.6^a

	Small		Large	
Group B	Water	Water	Water	Water
	13	5	12	7
	10	7	16	11
	14	18	6	5
	13	13	13	12
	21	6	19	8
	6	3	18	6
	15	13	15	2
Mean:	13.1	9.3	14.1	7.3

	Small Alcohol 700 mg.%	Large Alcohol 700 mg.%
Group C		
	8	30
	5	30
	20	30
	12	30
	8	30
	16	22
	22	30
Mean:	13	28.8^b

[a] P < .01

[b] P < .005

memory fixation, a level of 700 mg% might still induce a strong alcohol-amnesia. Therefore, we believe that changing the neurochemical substrate might be a good strategy for attempts to dissociate effects on rate of learning from possible effects on the later consolidation stage of memory formation.

CONCLUDING REMARKS

We have briefly reviewed some prominent symptoms of alcohol intoxication in humans (amnesia, state-dependent learning, and enhancement phenomena) and have found that these can be found in the behavior of goldfish as well. The most parsimonious hypothesis regarding the neural locus of alcohol's effects on memory is that disruption of mesencephalic or diencephalic systems (which includes corticofugal effects on these loci) could account for impairment of memory during high alcohol levels in fish or mammal. It can be hypothesized that probing the CNS for physiological or neurochemical correlates of memory is easier in the small fish brain than in the mammal, but interpretations from such studies will generalize in large part to the mammalian brain. The success enjoyed by Shashoua in measuring subtle shifts in RNA or protein metabolism during learning encourages us in our optimism concerning the goldfish model. The studies of Heiligenberg (1975) suggest that motivational systems can also be titrated with great sensitivity in fish such that a "neurochemistry of affect" can also be pursued with success at this phylogenetic level. These studies fully support our basic premise that a biological analysis for pervasive behavioral phenomena should always include the simplest organisms in which the behavior in question is already well developed.

ACKNOWLEDGMENTS

I would like to thank Mr. Mark Sostek, Dr. Marsha Vannicelli, and Dr. David Ingle for their help in completing this manuscript. The study discussed starting on p. 14 was supported in part by General Research Support Grant FR05484.

REFERENCES

Adams, R. A. The anatomy of memory mechanisms in the human brain. In G. A. Talland & N. C. Waugh (Eds.), *The pathology of memory*. New York: Academic Press, 1969.

Agranoff, B. W. Agents that block memory. In G. C. Quarton, T. Melnechuk, & F. O Schmitt (Eds.), *The neurosciences*. New York: Rockefeller University Press, 1967.

Agranoff, B. W., & Klinger, P. D. Puromycin effect on memory fixation in the goldfish. *Science*, 1964, *146*, 952–953.

Bernstein, J. J. Brightness discrimination following forebrain ablation in fish. *Experimental neurology*, 1961, *3*, 297–306.

Bernstein, J. J. Anatomy and physiology of the central nervous system. In W. S. Hoar & D. J. Randall (Eds.), *Fish physiology* (Vol. 4). New York: Academic Press, 1970.

Bitterman, M. E. Thorndike and the problem of animal intelligence. *American Psychologist,* 1969, *24,* 444–453.

Bryant, R. C., Petty, F., Warren, J. L., & Byrne, W. L. Facilitation by alcohol of active avoidance acquisition performance in the goldfish. *Pharmacology, Biochemistry and Behavior,* 1973, *1,* 523–529.

Butters, N., & Cermak, L. Some analysis of amnesic syndrome in brain-damaged patients. In R. L. Isaacson & K. H. Pribram (Eds.), *The hippocampus* (Vol. 2). New York: Plenum Press, 1975.

Carpenter, J. A., Moore, O. K., Snyder, C. R., & Lisansky, E. S. Alcohol and higher-order problem solving. *Quarterly Journal of Studies on Alcohol,* 1961, *22,* 183–222.

Carpenter, J. A., & Ross, B. M. Effect of alcohol on short-term memory. *Quarterly Journal of Studies on Alcohol,* 1965, *26,* 561–579.

Cermak, L. S., & Butters, N. The role of interference and encoding in the short-term memory deficits of Korsakoff patients. *Neuropsychologia,* 1972, *10,* 89–95.

Cermak, L. S., & Butters, N., & Gerrein, J. The extent of verbal encoding ability of Korsakoff patients. *Neuropsychologia,* 1973, *11,* 85–94.

Cermak, L. S., & Ryback, R. S. Recovery of verbal short-term memory in alcoholics. *Journal of Studies on Alcohol,* 1976, *37,* 46–52.

Crow, L. T. Effects of alcohol on conditioned avoidance responding. *Physiology and Behavior,* 1966, *1,* 89–91.

Demski, L., & Knigₑe, K. M. The telencephalon and hypothalamus of the Bluegill (Lepomis machrochirus): Evoked feeding, aggressive and reproductive behavior with representative frontal sections. *Journal of Comparative Neurology,* 1971, *143,* 1–16.

Diethelm, O., & Barr, R. M. Experimental study of amnesic periods in acute alcohol intoxication. *Psychiatria et Neurologia* (Basel), 1962, *144,* 5–14. (a)

Diethelm, O., & Barr, R. M. Psychotherapeutic interviews and alcohol intoxication. *Quarterly Journal of Studies on Alcohol,* 1962, *23,* 243–251. (b)

Ebbesson, S. O. E. A proposal for a common nomenclature for some optic nuclei in vertebrates and the evidence for a common origin of two such cell groups. *Brain, Behavior and Evolution,* 1972, *6,* 75–91.

Goodwin, D. W., Crane, J. B., & Guze, S. B. Alcoholic "blackouts": A review and clinical study of 100 alcoholics. *American Journal of Psychiatry,* 1969, *126,* 191–198. (a)

Goodwin, D. W., Othmer, E., Halikas, J. A., & Freemon, F. Loss of short-term memory as a predictor of the alcoholic "blackout" *Nature,* 1970, *227,* 201–202.

Goodwin, D. W., Powell, B., Bremer, D., Hoine, H., & Stern, J. Alcohol and recall: State-dependent effects in man. *Science,* 1969, *163,* 1358–1360. (b)

Heber, G., & Kryspin–Exner, K. Experimentelle Untersuchungen zur Frage der sogenannten Palimpseste bei Alkoholkranken. *Wierner Zietschrift fur Nervenheilkunde,* 1966, *24,* 219–226.

Heiligenberg, W. Analysis of mood and aggression in fish. *In* D. Ingle & H. M. Shein (Eds.), *Model systems in biological psychiatry.* Cambridge, Mass.: M. I. T. Press, 1975.

Holloway, F. A. State-dependent effects of ethanol on active and passive avoidance learning. *Psychopharmacologia,* 1972, *25,* 238–261.

Hutchinson, H. W., Tuchtie, M., Gray, K. G., & Steinberg, D. A study of the effects of alcohol on mental functions. *Canadian Psychiatric Association Journal,* 1964, *9,* 33–42.

Illchysin, D., & Ryback, R. S. Short-term memory in non-intoxicated alcoholics as a function of blackout history. Presented at Annual Conference of the National Council on Alcoholism, Washington, D.C., May 8, 1976; Ch. in F. A. Seixas (Ed.), *Currents in Alcoholism* (Vol. II). New York: Grune & Stratton, 1977.

Ingle, D. J. The use of the fish in neuropsychology. *Perspectives in Biology and Medicine,* 1965, *8,* 241–260. (a)

Ingle, D. J. Behavioral effects of forebrain lesions in goldfish. *Proceedings of the 73rd Annual Convention of the American Psychological Association,* 1965, 143–144. (b)

Ingle, D. Evolutionary perspectives on the function of the optic tectum. *Brain, Behavior and Evolution,* 1973, *8,* 211–237. (a)

Ingle, D. Reduction of habituation of prey catching activity by alcohol intoxication in the frog. *Behavioral Biology,* 1973, *8,* 123–129. (b)

Ingle, D. Enhancement of postrotary nystagmus by alcohol intoxication in the goldfish and in the frog. *Behavioral Biology,* 1973, *9,* 479–484. (c)

Jellinek, E. M. Phases in the drinking history of alcoholics: Analysis of a survey conducted by the official organ of Alcoholics Anonymous. *Quarterly Journal of Studies on Alcohol,* 1946, *7,* 1–8.

Jellinek, E. M. Phases of alcohol addiction. *Quarterly Journal of Studies on Alcohol,* 1952, *13,* 673–684.

Keller, M., & Seeley, J. R. *The alcohol language, with a selected vocabulary.* Toronto: University of Toronto Press, 1958.

Marshall, J. F., Turner, B. H., & Teitelbaum, P. Sensory neglect produced by lateral hypothalamic damage. *Science,* 1971, *174,* 523–525.

McGaugh, J. L. Memory storage processes. In K. H. Pribram & D. E. Broadbent (Eds.), *Biology of memory.* New York: Academic Press, 1970.

McNamee, H. B., Mello, N. K., & Mendelson, J. H. Experimental analysis of drinking patterns of alcoholics: Concurrent psychiatric observations. *American Journal of Psychiatry,* 1968, *124,* 1063–1069.

Mello, N. K. Short-term memory function in alcohol addicts during intoxication. In M. M. Gross (Ed.), *Alcohol intoxication and withdrawal: Experimental studies* (I.). New York: Plenum Press, 1973.

Milner, B. The memory defect in bilateral hippocampal lesions. *Psychiatric Research Reports of the American Psychiatric Association,* 1959, *11,* 43–58.

Moskowitz, H., & Murray, J. T. Alcohol and backward masking of visual information. *Journal of Studies on Alcohol,* 1976, *37,* 40–45.

Nash, H. *Alcohol and caffein: A study of their psychological effects.* Springfield, Ill.: C. C. Thomas, 1962.

Nolte, W. Experimentelle Untersuchungen zum Problem der Lokalisation des Assoziations vermogens im Fischgehirn. *Z. Vergl. Physiol.,* 1933, *18,* 255–279.

Olds, J., Disterhoft, J. F., & Segal, M. Learning centers of rat brain mapped by measuring latencies of conditioned unit responses. *Journal of Neurophysiology,* 1972, *35,* 202–219.

Overmier, J. B., & Savage, G. E. Effects of telencephalic ablation on trace classical condition of heart rate in goldfish. *Experimental Neurology,* 1974, *42,* 339–346.

Overton, D. A. State-dependent learning produced by depressant and atropine-like drugs. *Psychopharmacologia,* 1966, *10,* 6–31.

Overton, D. A. Discriminative control of behavior by drug states. In T. Thompson & R. Pickens (Eds.), *Stimulus properties of drugs.* New York: Appleton-Century-Crofts, 1971.

Peeke, H. V. S., Ellman, G. E., & Herz, M. J. Dose dependent alcohol effects on the aggressive behavior of the convict cichlid (*Cichlasoma nigrofasciatum*). *Behavioral Biology,* 1973, *8,* 115–122.

Petty, F., Bryant, R. C., & Byrne, W. L. Dose-related facilitation by alcohol of avoidance acquisition in the goldfish. *Pharmacology, Biochemistry and Behavior,* 1973, *1,* 173–176.

Pribram, K. H. The amnesic syndrome: Disturbance in coding. In G. A. Talland & N. C. Waugh (Eds.), *The pathology of memory.* New York: Academic Press, 1969.

Raynes, A. E., Ryback, R., & Ingle, D. The effect of alcohol on aggression in Betta Splendens. *Communication Behavioral Biology,* 1968, *2,* 141–146.

Regestein, Q. Some monocular emotional effects of unilateral hypothalamic lesions in goldfish. In D. Ingle (Ed.), *The central nervous system and fish behavior.* Chicago: University of Chicago Press, 1968.

Richardson, E. J. Alcohol-state dependent learning: Acquisition of a spatial discrimination in the goldfish (Carassius auratus). *Psychological Record,* 1972, *22,* 545–553.

Riege, W. H., & Cherkin, A. One-trial learning and biphasic time course of performance in the goldfish. *Science,* 1971, *172,* 966–968.

Ryback, R. S. The use of goldfish as a model for alcohol amnesia in man. *Quarterly Journal of Studies on Alcohol,* 1969, *30,* 877–882. (a)

Ryback, R. S. Effect of ethanol, bourbon and various ethanol levels on Y-maze learning in the goldfish. *Psychopharmacologia,* 1969, *14,* 305–314. (b)

Ryback, R. S. State-dependent or "dissociated" learning with alcohol in the goldfish. *Quarterly Journal of Studies on Alcohol,* 1969, *30,* 598–608. (c)

Ryback, R. S. Alcohol amnesia: Observations in seven inpatient drinking alcoholics. *Quarterly Journal of Studies on Alcohol,* 1970, *31,* 616–632. (a)

Ryback, R. S. The use of fish, especially goldfish, in alcohol research. *Quarterly Journal of Studies on Alcohol,* 1970, *31,* 162–166. (b)

Ryback, R. S. The continuum and specificity of the effects of alcohol on memory. A review. *Quarterly Journal of Studies on Alcohol,* 1971, *32,* 995–1016.

Ryback, R. S. Facilitation and inhibition of learning and memory by alcohol. *Annals of the New York Academy of Sciences,* 1973, *215,* 187–194.

Ryback, R. S. A method to study short-term memory (STM) in the goldfish. *Pharmacology Biochemistry and Behavior,* 1976, *4,* 489–491.

Ryback, R., Percarpio, B., & Vitale, J. Equilibration and metabolism of ethanol in the goldfish. *Nature,* 1969, *222,* 1068–1070.

Ryback, R. S., Weinert, J., & Fozard, J. L. Disruption of short-term memory in men following consumption of ethanol. *Psychonomic Science,* 1970, *20,* 353–354.

Sakitt, B. Locus of short-term visual storage. *Science,* 1975, *190,* 1318–1319.

Savage, G. E., & Swingland, I. R. Positively reinforced behaviour and the forebrain in goldfish. *Nature,* 1969, *221,* 878–879.

Schnitzlein, H. N. Introductory remarks on the telencephalon of fish. In D. Ingle (Ed.), *The central nervous system and fish behavior.* Chicago: University of Chicago Press, 1968.

Schulman, S. Impairment in delayed response following bilateral destruction of the dorsomedial nucleus of the thalamus in Rhesus monkeys. *Transactions of the American Neurological Association,* 1964, *89,* 122–125.

Scobie, S. R., & Bliss, D. K. Ethyl alcohol: Relationships to memory for aversive learning in goldfish (Carassius auratus). *Journal of Comparative and Physiological Psychology,* 1974, *86,* 867–874.

Shashoua, V. E. RNA changes in goldfish brain during learning. *Nature,* 1968, *217,* 238–240.

Shashoua, V. E. RNA metabolism of goldfish brain during acquisition of new behavioral patterns. *Proceedings of the National Academy of Sciences,* 1970, *65,* 160–162.

Shashoua, V. E. The goldfish as a model experimental animal for studies of biochemical correlates of the information storage process. In D. J. Ingle & I. M. Shein (Eds.), *Model systems in biological psychiatry.* Cambridge, Mass.: M. I. T. Press, 1975.

Sheer, D. E. Electrophysiological correlates of memory consolidation. In G. Ungar (Ed.), *Molecular mechanisms in memory and learning.* New York: Plenum Press, 1970.

Shupe, L. Alcohol and crime. A study of the urine alcohol concentrations found in 882 persons arrested during or immediately after the commission of a felony. *Journal of Criminal Law, Criminology and Police Science,* 1954, *44,* 661–664.

Shuttleworth, E. C., & Morris, C. E. The transient global amnesia syndrome: A defect in the second stage of memory in man. *Archives of Neurology,* 1966, *15,* 515–520.

Sperling, G. The information available in brief visual presentation. *Psychological Monographs,* 1960, *74,* (11, Whole No. 498).

Storm, T., & Caird, W. K. The effects of alcohol on serial verbal learning in chronic alcoholics. *Psychonomic Science,* 1967, *9,* 43–44.

Tamerin, J. S., Weiner, S., Poppen, R., Steinglass, P., & Mendelson, J. H. Alcohol and memory: Amnesia and short-term memory function during experimentally induced intoxication. *American Journal of Psychiatry,* 1971, *127,* 1659–1664.

Wallgren, H., & Barry, H., III. *Actions of alcohol* (Vol. 2). New York: Elsevier Publishing Co., 1970.

Warrington, E. K., & Weiskrantz, L. An analysis of short-term and long-term memory defects in man. In J. A. Deutsch (Ed.), *The physiological basis of memory.* New York: Academic Press, 1973.

Washburne, C. Alcohol, amnesia and awareness. *Quarterly Journal of Studies on Alcohol,* 1958, *19,* 471–481.

9
Alcohol and Memory Impairment in Male and Female Social Drinkers

Ben Morgan Jones
Marilyn K. Jones

Oklahoma Center for Alcohol and Drug Related Studies,
Department of Psychiatry and Behavioral Sciences
The University of Oklahoma Health Sciences Center

INTRODUCTION

The influence of alcohol on human memory has received considerable attention during the last few years (Ryback, 1971; Jones, 1973; Parker, Alkana, Birnbaum, Hartley, & Noble, 1974; Wickelgren, 1975; Moskowitz & Murray, 1976; Weingartner, Adefris, Eich, & Murphy, 1976). Although impaired memory ability following acute alcohol ingestion may be one of the most common and reproducible effects reported by social drinkers, there has been surprisingly little systematic research investigating the variables that influence this memory deficit and the theoretical nature of the impairment. This chapter will summarize a series of experiments using the free-recall technique to address three issues. The first issue concerns the relationship of memory impairment to the alcohol dose and to the direction of change of the blood alcohol level during a particular testing session. Larger alcohol doses may produce greater memory impairment for certain type of memory functions. Memory also may be more impaired while the blood-alcohol level is increasing than while it is decreasing for a given dose. Therefore, it may not be sufficient to report only the blood alcohol level at the time of testing. Quantitative as well as possible qualitative memory differences on the ascending and descending limbs of the blood-alcohol curve also might aid in the interpretation of the nature of the alcohol-induced memory impairment.

The second issue revolves around the nature of the memory impairment in terms of the retrieval vs. consolidation type of deficits. It appears important to determine whether the information is available under the influence of alcohol but cannot be adequately retrieved or whether alcohol interferes with the consolidation of memory traces such that the information is not permanently stored. If retrieval is impaired by alcohol, then certain procedures might be developed to assist in recall. However, if consolidation is impaired, then it may be virtually impossible for an individual to recall certain types of information learned under the influence of alcohol. Procedures might then be developed to assist in the organization of material that might aid in the consolidation of information under the influence of alcohol.

The third issue is related to possible differences in the effects of alcohol on memory in male and female social drinkers. The majority of data evaluating the effects of alcohol on memory have been obtained from male social drinkers. Since it has been suggested that cognitive abilities in males and females may be differentially affected by certain types of drugs (Broverman, Klaiber, Kobayashi, & Vogel, 1968), it appears appropriate to determine if alcohol affects memory processes differentially in males and females. This is especially important, since females comprise approximately the same number of social drinkers as males in our society. Differences in the effect of alcohol on memory in males and females also might aid in determining possible influences of the sex hormones on memory ability. For instance, it has been suggested that low sex-hormonal levels result in greater alcohol effects in animals (Goldberg & Stortebecker, 1943). It also has been reported that high levels of sex hormones may increase performance on certain types of cognitive tasks (Klaiber, Broverman, Vogel & Mackenberg, 1974).

We have conducted several memory studies using a free-recall verbal-memory task. Since the general procedures for these studies were virtually identical, we will outline our procedure first and then go on to discuss the results of the studies. There are a number of methodological considerations that are critical for research on the acute effects of alcohol. We hope to highlight some of them by a somewhat detailed presentation of the methods employed in our laboratory.

METHOD

Subjects. All subjects in the studies to be reported were paid volunteer, moderate social drinkers. The subjects all had a high school degree, and most had some college (the range was 12 to 19 years of education). The mean age of our subjects was 25 years with a range from 21 to 34 years. The subjects in the first studies were all males, whereas subjects in later studies were both males and females. Male and female data were reported and analyzed separately. Subjects were instructed to obtain a regular night's sleep prior to the testing days and not to drink alcoholic beverages or take any medication or drugs the night prior to testing or on the day of testing. Subjects were asked to eat a light breakfast about 9:00 A.M. on the day of testing and not to eat, drink, or smoke from that time until reporting to the laboratory at 12:00 noon. Subjects remained in the laboratory until they obtained a zero blood alcohol level, and then were escorted home after the completion of testing.

Alcohol concentration. Subjects first read and signed a human consent form approved by the Human Experimentation Committee. Subjects were then weighed, and those in the low-dose group received 0.52g 95% USP ethanol per kilogram of body weight (0.52g/kg); and subjects in the high-dose group received 1.04g 95% USP ethanol per kilogram of body weight (1.04g/kg). The alcohol was mixed with orange drink in the ratio of 4:1 — four parts orange drink to one part ethanol for both doses. The low dose resulted in a peak blood alcohol level of about 0.06%, and the high dose resulted in a peak blood alcohol level of about 0.11% for the male subjects. Slightly higher levels were obtained for the females. Placebo subjects received the same volume drink as the high-dose alcohol subjects with only four milliliters of ethanol floated on top of the orange drink to provide an alcohol taste. The subjects in the low-dose group were paced so that they consumed the drink in exactly 5 minutes; subjects in the high-dose group were paced so they consumed their drink in exactly 15 minutes. Drinking time was strictly controlled, since it has been reported that drinking time is related to cognitive performance (Jones & Vega, 1973; Moskowitz & Burns, 1976). The low-alcohol dose was equivalent to 3 ounces of 95-proof liquor for a 150-pound person, or about 2 to 3 mixed drinks. The high-alcohol dose was equivalent to 6 ounces of 95-proof liquor for a 150-pound person, or about 4 to 6 mixed drinks (Jones & Jones, 1976b).

Breathalyzer samples. It has been only in the last few years that it has become practical to measure the blood alcohol level and have the results available in a few minutes so that a subject could be tested at a specific blood alcohol level. Our general procedure was to take a practice breath on a Breathalyzer (Stephenson Model 900) or an Intoxilyzer (Omicron, Model 4011) prior to drinking to insure that subjects had a zero blood alcohol level prior to drinking. All subjects registered zero on the practice breath. Immediately after the subjects finished drinking, they rinsed their mouth with water to clear it of residual alcohol. Breath samples were taken about every 5 minutes, until the subject reached the peak blood alcohol level, and every 5 to 10 minutes thereafter on the descending limb. High correlations between breath analysis samples and direct blood analyses ($r = 0.956$) have been reported in several recent reviews of the validity and reliability of breath measurement (Dubowski, 1970, 1975). The first two or three breath readings usually were invalid (too high, due to residual alcohol in the mouth and throat). Valid breath readings were obtained about 10 to 15 minutes after the end of drinking, which is in agreement with other reports (Jones, 1973; Jones & Jones, 1976a; Spector, 1971; Dubowski, 1975). The four milliliters of alcohol given to the placebo subjects did not produce a detectable reading on the Breathalyzer. Breath samples also were taken immediately before the beginning of the memory task, in the middle of the task, and at the end of the task for both alcohol and placebo subjects. An average of about 25 breath samples was obtained on each subject.

Memory task. The subjects were tested on a free-recall verbal memory task as described by Glanzer (1971). A total of 216 monosyllabic high-frequency nouns were drawn from the Thorndike-Lorge (1944) AA lists and randomly assigned to 18 lists with 12 words per list. Each word was printed in black on a white background with one word per slide. The words were displayed on a screen with a 35-millimeter Carousel projector. Each slide was on for 1 second with a 1-second interval between slides. The screen was approximately 3 feet from the subject. Total time for each list was 24 seconds. The subjects read each word aloud and then started writing words immediately after termination of the 12th word. The subjects were allowed a 1-minute free-recall period to write their responses. The next list was presented 30 seconds after responses to the previous list were obtained.

A block diagram of the procedure is presented in Figure 1. The 18 lists were divided into 3 groups of 6 lists per group. Group-1 lists were presented to subjects before alcohol to obtain baseline measures for immediate and short-term memory. The immediate-memory score was the total words correct for the individual recall of each of the 6 lists (72 possible). Thirty seconds after recall of the 6th list, subjects were given 5 minutes to recall words from all 6 lists in any order. This was the short-term memory score. The drinking period immediately followed the baseline short-term memory task. Subjects in the low-dose group were given group-2 lists when they reached 0.04% on the ascending limb and group-3 lists after they reached peak and were at 0.04% on the descending limb of the blood alcohol curve. Subjects in the high-dose group were tested at 0.09% on the ascending limb and 0.09% on the descending limb. Immediate and short-term memory scores were obtained at both times. The placebo group was tested at three times similar to the alcohol groups.

Subjects also were administered the Shipley Institute of Living Scale and the Eysenck Personality Inventory before alcohol to assess basic intelligence and personality variables respectively.

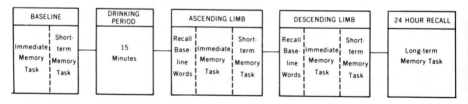

FIGURE 1   Block diagram of the procedure (see below). (From Jones, 1973. Copyright 1973 by the American Psychological Association. Reprinted by permission.)

ASCENDING—DESCENDING LIMB EFFECTS

The direction of change of the blood alcohol level has been reported to be a significant variable in evaluating both behavioral and psychological changes following acute alcohol ingestion (Jones, Parsons, & Rundell, 1976). The basic finding in the literature is that performance is more impaired on the ascending limb (increasing blood alcohol level) than on the descending limb (decreasing blood alcohol level) at comparable blood alcohol levels. These results suggest that the effects of alcohol on memory should be evaluated not only at specific blood alcohol levels but also on the ascending and descending limbs of the blood alcohol curve to adequately interpret the effect of alcohol on memory. The data to be summarized below were originally published by Jones (1973) for the high-dose and placebo groups and by Jones and Jones (1976a) for the low-dose group. However, since the testing conditions were equivalent for both studies, the results were combined for the purpose of comparison in this chapter.

Immediate memory. The data for the placebo, low-dose, and high-dose groups for immediate memory are presented in Table 1. An overall alcohol effect was obtained for both low and high dose compared to baseline performance of each group. A comparison of ascending limb and descending limb alcohol performances with the placebo group performance also was significant. Although the placebo group improved slightly from first to third group of words, this difference was not statistically significant. A comparison of ascending and descending performances indicated that descending limb performance was significantly better than ascending limb performance for both the low and the high-alcohol-dose groups.

Short-term memory. Mean scores for short-term memory for the three groups also are presented in Table 1. An overall alcohol effect was found for both the

TABLE 1

Mean (± S.E.) Scores for Immediate and Short-Term Memory for Placebo, Low-Dose (0.52 g/kg), and High-Dose (1.04 g/kg) Alcohol Groups (Males) Tested During Baseline and on the Ascending and Descending Limbs of the Blood Alcohol Curve.

	Baseline	Ascending limb	Descending limb
Immediate memory			
1. Placebo (N = 20) −0.00%	41.60 ± 1.50	42.65 ± 1.74	43.65 ± 1.81
2. Low dose (N = 10) −0.04%	39.00 ± 2.92	32.50 ± 2.37	36.40 ± 2.83
3. High dose (N = 20) −0.09%	43.45 ± 1.97	35.25 ± 1.75	38.30 ± 1.97
Short-term memory			
1. Placebo (N = 20) −0.00%	19.00 ± 1.31	19.00 ± 2.07	20.45 ± 2.25
2. Low dose (N = 10) −0.04%	20.70 ± 2.77	11.80 ± 2.24	12.60 ± 2.33
3. High dose (N = 20) −0.09%	20.50 ± 1.75	6.70 ± 1.02	7.50± 1.04

low- and high-alcohol-dose groups. However, there were no significant differences between ascending and descending limb performances for either alcohol group. It also is clear that the effect of alcohol is greater for short-term memory than for immediate memory.

These results clearly demonstrate that ascending—descending limb differences should be considered in examining the effects of alcohol on memory. Immediate memory was consistently more impaired on the ascending than on the descending limb. However, short-term memory, which was more impaired by alcohol than immediate memory, did not demonstrate an ascending—descending limb difference. It should be noted that there was no dose-response relationship for alcohol on the immediate-memory task. Both low- and high-alcohol-dose groups showed similar impairment. However, a dose-response relationship was found for the short-term memory task as presented in Table 1. These results point out that these two types of memory may be differentially affected by alcohol.

RETRIEVAL VS. CONSOLIDATION DEFICITS

The memory deficits due to alcohol may be due to poor retrieval of information or failure of the information to be properly consolidated into long-term memory. It has been reported that severe memory deficits due to alcohol ingestion — blackouts — usually occur during the time of rapidly rising blood alcohol levels (Ryback, 1971). Since blackouts appear to be a result of failure of consolidation of events and occur on the ascending limb, it may be that memory deficits at the low blood-alcohol levels we have reported may be more likely to be due to consolidation deficits.

One method of evaluating the locus of the memory deficit in the free-recall task is to examine the serial position curves. The typical finding in a nondrug state is that the subject recalls words better from the beginning of the list (primacy effect) and the end of the list (recency effect) than from the middle of the list. There have been a variety of explanations for this effect. Glanzer (1971) has proposed one explanation that appears to be relevant in interpreting the effect of alcohol on memory. Glanzer presents data that is compatible with his contention that the last few words can be recalled easily and go into short-term storage (STS). However, these words are easily forgotten and are replaced by new words. Words in the first positions of a list also are easily recalled, but these words are in long-term storage and are not easily displaced by new words. These words from the first part of a list would then be expected to make up short-term memory. Since alcohol dramatically affected short-term memory, it is possible that alcohol may selectively impair recall of words from the first positions of the list (LTS) while not significantly affecting recall of words from the end of the lists (STS). If alcohol does impair recall of words more from LTS than from STS, then this provides some support that retrieval may not be impaired. If,

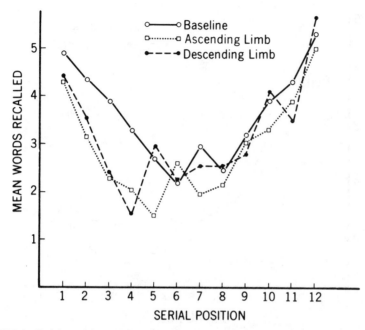

FIGURE 2 Serial position curves for the immediate-memory task for the high-dose (1.04g/kg) alcohol group (see below). (From Jones, 1973. Copyright 1973 by the American Psychological Association. Reprinted by permission.)

however, recall is impaired equally from all serial positions, then this would provide support that alcohol does, indeed, interfere with retrieval of the words. Since the major affect of alcohol was found on the ascending limb, the majority of the results reported will be for the ascending limb data, although similar results were found for the descending limb.

Serial position curves for immediate memory for the high alcohol dose are presented in Figure 2. Similar results were obtained with the low-alcohol-dose group (Jones & Jones, 1976c). It is clear from Figure 2 that alcohol does not produce an overall decrease in recall from all serial positions. An interaction of recall with serial position was found in that alcohol reduced recall of words from the first part of each list (LTS) but not from the last positions (STS). These data suggest that retrieval per se cannot account for this effect. It also supports the finding that alcohol impairs short-term memory, since most of the words recalled in short-term memory usually are words from the first positions of each list (LTS). The serial position curves for short-term memory are illustrated in Figure 3. Recall of baseline words do come primarily from the first three to four positions in each list, with fewer words coming from the last positions. However, alcohol decreased the recall from these first positions as might be expected. Thus, a flat and somewhat linear curve was found for the alcohol condition.

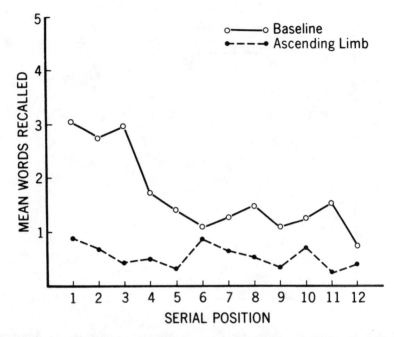

FIGURE 3   Serial position curves for the short-term memory task for the high-dose (1.04g/kg) alcohol group (see below). (From Jones, 1973. Copyright 1973 by the American Psychological Association. Reprinted by permission.)

These data also suggest that recall of words presented to the subject under the influence of alcohol was not impaired equally across all serial positions and retrieval deficits cannot explain the results. The greatest impairment was for words thought to be consolidated into long-term memory.

However, it could be argued that for some reason alcohol selectively impaired retrieval of words in the first positions of a list while not impairing retrieval of words from other positions. This possibility was examined by analyzing the recall of baseline words during the alcohol state. Subjects were asked to recall baseline words on the ascending limb after they had completed the ascending limb memory tasks. It was found that the decrease in recall of baseline words from baseline to ascending limb was not any greater than decrease in the placebo group. These results indicated that the presence of alcohol did not interfere with retrieval of words seen before alcohol, indicating that retrieval per se could not explain the alcohol deficits. The serial position curve for recall of baseline words during alcohol was similar to recall during baseline, indicating that the presence of alcohol does not prevent retrieval per se but does appear to interfere with the proper consolidation and storage of information.

It still might be argued that the words are really properly consolidated and stored and that they could be adequately retrieved if the subjects were exposed to the same material a second or third time. Data from repeated exposure to the same words for three testing sessions approximately 1 week apart are currently being collected for males and females tested on the low dose (0.52g/kg). Baseline performance appears to improve about twice that of alcohol performance. Most of the improvement for the alcohol condition occurs from first to second session. However, a greater alcohol impairment appears from session to session since baseline performance continues to improve. Serial position curves for baseline performance for first and third sessions show a general improvement for all serial positions. The effect of practice during the alcohol condition was to selectively improve recall from the last positions (STS) but not from the first positions (LTS). Serial position curves for short-term memory for baseline indicate an improvement across all positions. Serial position curves for ascending limb performance for the first and third sessions indicate there is no increase in recall of words from the first positions but there is an increase in recall of words in the last positions. These results from the practice effects indicate that repeated practice did not result in greater recall of words from LTS and indicated that the alcohol-induced deficit is probably not a result of impaired retrieval mechanisms.

An analysis of the effect of practice on the recall of baseline words during alcohol indicated that practice improved recall of these words to about the same extent as recall during baseline. Again, retrieval of baseline words was not impaired during alcohol. Improvement in recall of words from the first positions also was found. However, this same improvement was not found in words presented and recalled during alcohol, suggesting that alcohol selectively interferes with the consolidation of words into short-term memory and does not greatly affect retrieval of words.

MALE VS. FEMALE SOCIAL DRINKERS

The data reported up to this point were collected on male social drinkers. It appeared possible that the effects of alcohol might be different for females than for males. We have found that females obtain significantly higher peak blood alcohol levels than males on the same alcohol dose, calculated on total body weight. We also have found differences in males and females in absorption and elimination rates (Jones & Jones, 1976a). It has been reported by others that males and females may perform differently on certain cognitive tasks and that certain drugs may differentially affect performance of males and females (Broverman, Klaiber, Kobayashi, & Vogel, 1968). The present study was directed at determining whether alcohol affects memory of females differently than males.

We tested a group of 20 women and 10 men in our first study on the free-recall task on the low dose of 0.04% on the ascending and descending limbs of the blood alcohol curves. There were no significant differences in baseline performances for the immediate- or short-term memory scores. Also, the effect of alcohol on immediate memory was similar for both groups. However, we found that the females were significantly more affected than males by alcohol on the short-term memory task. These data indicate that alcohol may affect females to a greater extent than males on tasks that require a delayed response. A more detailed study is now being conducted to examine the effects of alcohol at different times during the menstrual cycle. We also are testing women who are taking oral contraceptives to determine if alcohol interacts with synthetic hormones to produce different memory effects.

The women in our ongoing study are tested during the menstrual phase, the intermenstrual phase and the premenstrual phase in a counterbalanced order. Although this study is still in progress, some preliminary findings will be mentioned. First an analysis by sessions indicates that both groups of females are affected by alcohol in a similar manner to males for the immediate-memory task. One difference between the two female groups is that the women taking oral contraceptives did not show a significant ascending–descending limb effect for immediate or short-term memory for any of the three sessions. The women also were more impaired by alcohol than the men on short-term memory for the first session. However, this difference disappeared with practice on the second and third sessions.

Preliminary data for the women tested with respect to the phase of the menstrual cycle also are being collected. These data should be interpreted cautiously since some of the differences may be attributed to practice effects at this point. In general, baseline performance was the poorest during the intermenstrual phase for both immediate and short-term memory. The largest effects of alcohol occurred during the menstrual and the premenstrual phases for both memory measures. These differences suggest that alcohol may have a greater effect on memory in women during times of low hormonal levels. More detailed analyses of these data are currently in progress.

SUMMARY

Data from our laboratory suggest that alcohol impairs both immediate and short-term memory as assessed by a free-recall verbal memory task. Immediate memory is more impaired on the ascending than on the descending limb of the blood alcohol curve at both high and low doses. Practice appears to enhance the effect of alcohol on both immediate and short-term memory, mainly because practice results in a greater increase in recall for baseline than alcohol words. The effects of alcohol as a function of serial position provide some evidence that the alcohol deficits may not be attributable to impaired retrieval per se, but the deficits appear to be more consistent with an impaired consolidation and storage of information. Males and females demonstrated similar baseline memory performance, but alcohol produced a greater impairment in short-term memory scores for females. Preliminary data also indicated that alcohol may have a greater effect on memory when women are tested during the menstrual or premenstrual phase of their menstrual cycle as compared to the intermenstrual phase. Women taking oral contraceptives were similar to women not taking oral contraceptives on the memory scores, except that women taking the pill did not demonstrate ascending–descending limb differences. The finding that even relatively small doses of alcohol can produce rather pronounced and consistent memory impairment has implications for moderate use of alcohol by social drinkers.

ACKNOWLEDGMENTS

We would like to express our appreciation to Millie Kratina for the typing of the manuscript and to John Farris and Elizabeth Hatcher for testing of the subjects and data analysis.

This research was supported in part by Public Health Service Grant R01 AA01444 from the National Institute on Alcohol Abuse and Alcoholism entitled "Effects of Alcohol on Women During the Menstrual Cycle" under the direction of Ben Morgan Jones, Ph.D.

REFERENCES

Broverman, D. M., Klaiber, E. L., Kobayashi, Y., & Vogel, W. Roles of activation and inhibition in sex differences in cognitive abilities. *Psychological Review,* 1968, *75,* 23–50.

Dubowski, K. M. Measurement of ethyl alcohol in breath. In F. W. Sunderman & F. W. Sunderman, Jr. (Eds.), *Laboratory diagnosis of diseases caused by toxic agents.* St. Louis, Missouri: Warren H. Green, 1970.

Dubowski, K. M. Studies in breath-alcohol analysis: Biological factors. *Zeitschrift fur Rechtsmedizin,* 1975, *76,* 93–117.

Glanzer, M. Short-term storage and long-term storage in recall. *Journal of Psychiatric Research,* 1971, *8,* 423–438.

Goldberg, L., & Stortebecker, T. P. The antinarcotic effect of estrone on alcohol intoxication. *Acta Physiologica Scandinavica,* 1943, *5,* 289–296.

Jones, B. M. Memory impairment on the ascending and descending limbs of the blood alcohol curve. *Journal of Abnormal Psychology,* 1973, *82,* 24–32.

Jones, B. M., & Jones, M. K. Alcohol effects in women during the menstrual cycle. *Annals of the New York Academy of Sciences,* 1976, *273,* 576–587. (a)

Jones, B. M., & Jones, M. K. Male and female intoxication levels for three doses or do women really get higher than men? *Alcohol Technical Reports,* 1976, *5,* 11–14. (b)

Jones, B. M., & Jones, M. K. Women and alcohol: Intoxication, metabolism, and the menstrual cycle. In M. Greenblatt & M. A. Schuckit (Eds.), *Alcoholism problems in women and children.* New York: Grune & Stratton, 1976. (c)

Jones, B. M., Parsons, O. A., & Rundell, O. H. Psychophysiological correlates of alcoholism. In R. E. Tarter & A. A. Sugerman (Eds.), *Alcoholism: interdisciplinary approaches to an enduring problem.* Reading, Mass.: Addison-Wesley, 1976.

Jones, B. M., & Vega, A. Fast and slow drinkers: Blood alcohol variables and cognitive performance. *Quarterly Journal of Studies on Alcohol,* 1973, *34,* 797–806.

Klaiber, E. L., Broverman, D. M., Vogel, W., & Mackenberg, E. J. Rhythms in cognitive functioning and EEG indices in males. In M. Ferin, F. Holberg, R. M. Richart, & R. L. Vande Wiele (Eds.), *Biorhythms and human reproduction.* New York: Wiley, 1974.

Moskowitz, H., and Burns, M. Effects of rate of drinking on human performance. *Journal of Studies on Alcohol,* 1976, *37,* 598–605.

Moskowitz, H., & Murray, J. T. Alcohol and backward masking of visual information. *Journal of Studies on Alcohol,* 1976, *37,* 40–45.

Parker, E. S., Alkana, R. L., Birnbaum, I. M., Hartley, J. T., & Noble, E. P. Alcohol and the disruption of cognitive processes. *Archives of General Psychiatry,* 1974, *31,* 824–828.

Ryback, R. S. The continuum and specificity of the effects of alcohol on memory: A review. *Quarterly Journal of Studies on Alcohol,* 1971, *32,* 995–1016.

Spector, N. H. Alcohol breath tests: Gross errors in current methods of measuring alveolar gas concentrations. *Science,* 1971, *172,* 57–59.

Thorndike, E. L., & Lorge, I. *The teacher's book of 30,000 words.* New York: Columbia University, Teachers College Press, 1944.

Weingartner, H., Adefris, W., Eich, J. E., & Murphy, D. L. Encoding-imagery specificity in alcohol state-dependent learning. *Journal of Experimental Psychology: Human Learning and Memory,* 1976, *2,* 83–87.

Wickelgren, W. A. Alcoholic intoxication and memory storage dynamics. *Memory & Cognition,* 1975, *3,* 385–389.

Part IV

ALCOHOL
AND STATE DEPENDENCY

10
State-Dependent Retrieval of Information in Human Episodic Memory

James Eric Eich

University of Toronto and
National Institute of Mental Health

Utilization or retrieval of information in human episodic memory (Tulving, 1972) depends in part for its success on the drug-induced state of the individual at the time of (a) encoding and storage of the information and (b) its attempted utilization. A person asked to remember a simple event such as the appearance of a familiar word in an otherwise unfamiliar list or collection of other words, typically shows impaired retrieval for the word-event when his state is changed between the study and test sessions of the experiment, in comparison with conditions where his state remains the same on both occasions. This interaction of drug states at study and at test defines a phenomenon of human memory that customarily is referred to as *dissociated* or *state-dependent learning*. But since it is clearly the congruence of drug states present at study and at test that is responsible for the phenomenon (Melton, 1963; Tulving, 1968), state-dependent *retrieval* or *utilization* of information about the occurrence of perceptual episodes or events would seem to be a more appropriate expression (Wickelgren, 1975).

Human state-dependent retrieval (SDR) has been a focus of experimental investigation for only about 10 years. In that time a good deal has been learned about the form, if not the substance, of SDR effects in man, though hardly everything one might want to know. Accordingly, it is the dual purpose of this chapter to review the evidence bearing on various aspects of the human SDR phenomenon and to point out some of the problems for which adequate solutions have not yet emerged. We will focus mainly on SDR induced by drugs and alcohol in particular; experimental studies of dissociative effects associated with disturbance of affect or mood have been reviewed elsewhere (Weingartner, 1977). Also, although the focus is on SDR as seen in "normal" adult humans, occasional reference will be made to studies in which either chronic alcoholics or hyperactive children participated as subjects, as well as to experimental work with animals. Finally, our attention will center on experimental studies in which either verbal or pictorial items — words, faces, nonsense syllables, geometric figures, and the like — serve as the foci of events about whose occurrence the subject's memory is tested. Dissociative effects of drugs upon autonomic responsivity, motor learning, or operant discriminative avoidance will not be reviewed here (see Crow & Ball, 1975; Hill, Schwin, Powell & Goodwin, 1973; Hinrichsen, Katahn, & Levenson, 1974; Ley, Jain, Swinson, Eaves, Bradshaw, Kincey, Crowder, & Abbiss, 1972; Overton, 1972).

The chapter is organized into four major sections. We begin with a brief discussion of some historical antecedents of the human SDR phenomenon. This is followed by a broadly stroked rendering of key empirical findings to date, together with discussion of some of the issues and problems currently of interest to students of human state dependence. The third section concerns the relation between the magnitude of SDR effects, on the one hand, and the nature or characteristics of the retrieval test, on the other. The final section details a brief prospectus on human SDR research, with particular emphasis on issues regarding the practical and clinical significance of the phenomenon.

Some Historical Antecedents

State-dependent retrieval is an anomaly among phenomena of human memory in that it was not so much discovered in the laboratory as it was simply confirmed. Long before the first set of relevant experimental data was subjected to an F test, there were at least three reasons for presupposing the occurrence of the phenomenon.

First, it had been known for a long time that how well an event is remembered depends, among other things, on the completeness of the reinstatement at recall of the context in which the event originally occurred. This "principle of reinstatement of stimulating conditions" (Hollingworth, 1928) has figured prominently in the writings of many contemporary memory theorists (e.g., Bower, 1972; Melton, 1963) and has been evinced in numerous experimental studies (see McGeoch, 1933).

Some students of human memory have found it useful to distinguish two or more senses of the term context (e.g., McGeoch, 1939; Reiff & Scheerer, 1959). One is the view of context as the totality of situational influences that emanate from without the experiencing organism. This category subsumes properties of the external environment such as the experimenter's voice, conceptual relations among to-be-remembered (target) words and corresponding retrieval cues (Light

& Carter–Sobell, 1970), the color of the laboratory's walls, and the like. A second meaning sometimes ascribed to context is the totality of situational influences arising from *within* the experiencing organism – influences that affect the way a person perceives, remembers, and thinks about the world, and which collectively represent the individual's internal or experiential context (Reiff & Scheerer, 1959). This was the sense of context early memory theorists had in mind when they spoke of perception and remembering being influenced by prevailing "attitude complexes" (Crosland, 1921), "sentiments" (Pear, 1922), and "psychic tension-systems" (Lewin, 1935). Clearly, this is also the sense of context aroused by the idea of a drug-altered state of mind, or brain. If we think of two readily discriminable drug states – call them states A and B – as representing different experiential contexts, then we may infer from the "reinstatement principle" that events experienced in state A may be more retrievable in state A than in state B. Analogously, events experienced in state B may be expected to be more accessible in the B state rather than the A state. This inference is by no means a recent theoretic insight. At the turn of the century, Richard Semon in his classic work *Die Mneme* (1904) wrote that "alcoholic intoxication may, under certain circumstances, create an energetic condition whose engrams are ecphorable [my translation: 'retrievable'] in the next state of intoxication, but not in the intervening state of sobriety [pp. 144–145]." In view of the apparent relation between the reinstatement principle on one hand and the concept of discriminable drug states on the other, recent experimental demonstrations of SDR effects in man seem neither counterintuitive nor surprising.

A second reason for anticipating the occurrence of dissociative effects in man was the fact that comparable effects had been observed in several animal species, using a variety of animal learning-tasks and with scores of centrally acting drugs. Drugs that exclusively act outside the central nervous system (CNS) do not produce dissociative effects in laboratory animals nor, perhaps, in man (Overton, 1968, 1971, 1973).

The third clue was the phenomenon of alcoholic blackout. It had been observed that alcoholics occasionally hide money or liquor while drinking, have no recollection of the hiding place while sober, but recapture the memory when again intoxicated (Goodwin, 1971; Goodwin, Powell, Bremer, Hoine, & Stern, 1969). Questions naturally arose as to whether these clinical impressions might be amenable to experimental scrutiny and whether an analogue of the alcoholic blackout might be found in nonalcoholic subjects.

Primarily in response to this last question, alcohol was used in several of the earliest (pre-1970) experimental studies of SDR effects in normal human adults, and it remains today the drug of choice for many investigators. Since the early 1970s, a modest but continuing effort has been made to determine the dissociative properties of other commonly used and frequently abused drugs (especially marijuana), and a few attempts have been made to demonstrate SDR using special-purpose, currently nonabused agents such as the cholinesterase inhibitor physostigmine. What these various researches have taught us about the phenomenon of human state-dependent retrieval is the focus of discussion in the next section of the chapter.

Current Findings and Issues

Most of the evidence that will be reviewed in this section comes from studies using a 2 × 2 factorial design, where two drug states at the time of encoding and storage of target events (the *study* session) are crossed with these same two states at retrieval (the *test* session). One state is defined in reference to the administration of a specific dose of a centrally acting drug; the other in reference to the administration of appropriate placebo material. The cross of the two factors defines the following four groups: (a) study drug-free, test drug-free (NN); (b) study drug-free, test drug (ND); (c) study drug, test drug-free (DN); and (d) study drug, test drug (DD). If the drug has a direct effect on the acquisition of information about target events (as, for example, by impairing encoding or consolidation processes), groups that study under drug will be deficient in test performance. By the same token, if the drug has a deleterious effect upon processes involved in the completion of the retention test, groups tested under drug will show impairment. Finally, if the drug produces a dissociative effect, then test performance (in most experimental situations) will be relatively poor in groups ND and DN; this is true since in these groups the drug states are different during the study and test sessions of the experiment. The degree to which test performance is impaired in these two groups relative to groups NN and DD, respectively, indicates the magnitude or robustness of the SDR effect (see Overton, 1972). Although the simultaneous occurrence of any two or all three of the aforementioned drug effects may make rigorous interpretation of the data rather difficult, the specific pattern of findings yielded by the 2 × 2 design, together with supplementary or pilot data, often will permit accurate analysis of the experimental results (Berger & Stein, 1969; Overton, 1972).

Drugs that produce SDR. One or more doses of six centrally acting drugs have been found to produce SDR effects in normal adult humans. These drugs and drug doses include:

1. approximately 0.7 to 1.2 g/kg absolute *alcohol*[1] (Crow & Ball, 1975; Goodwin et al., 1969; Tarter, 1970; Weingartner, Adefris, Eich, & Murphy, 1976; Weingartner, Eich, & Allen, 1973; Weingartner & Faillace, 1971);

---

[1] Two studies of the dissociative effects of alcohol will not be examined in this paper. One of these was conducted by Hinrichsen et al. (1974), who reported evidence of SDR using paired-associate learning procedures. Unfortunately, there are some problems with the

2. 200 mg of the barbiturate *amobarbital* (Bustamante, Jordán, Vila, González, & Insua, 1970; Bustamante, Rosselló, Jordán, Pradere, & Insua, 1968; Ley et al., 1972);

3. 20 mg of *d-amphetamine* (Bustamante et al., 1968, 1970);

4. the general anesthetic *isoflurane,* in end-tidal concentrations ranging from .01 to .64% (Adam, Castro, & Clark, 1974);

5. *marijuana* containing between 7.5 and 20.0 mg delta-9-tetrahydrocannabinol or THC (Darley, Tinklenberg, Roth, & Atkinson, 1974; Eich, Weingartner, Stillman, & Gillin, 1975; Hill et al., 1973; Rickles, Cohen, Whitaker, & McIntyre, 1973; Stillman, Weingartner, Wyatt, Gillin, & Eich, 1974);

6. 1 mg of the anticholinesterase agent *physostigmine* (Weingartner, 1977).

The nature of the relation between occurrence of SDR effects and drug dosage has not been systematically researched. What little evidence there is suggests that SDR is demonstrated most readily using moderate doses of the drugs listed above (see Overton, 1972). High doses of many centrally active drugs, particularly sedatives and anesthetics, often produce severe retention deficits that easily can obscure any dissociative effects that may be present. This is probably one reason why Osborn, Bunker, Cooper, Frank, and Hilgard (1967) found no evidence of SDR using a relatively high dose (2.5% aqueous solution, intravenous administration) of the anesthetic thiopental (see Overton, 1968, 1972). On the other hand, almost all the available evidence points to the conclusion that SDR effects occur only in conjunction with a significant main effect — facilitative or inhibitory — of drug on either acquisition or on test performance (see Swanson & Kinsbourne, 1976). Since neither main effect is likely to obtain given relatively low drug doses, it follows that light doses typically will fail to dissociate retrieval. It is important to note, however, that although a significant main effect of drug on acquisition or on test performance may be a necessary condition for the demonstration of SDR, such an effect does not represent a sufficient condition. As we will see shortly, the occurrence of SDR effects critically depends, among other things, on the nature of the retrieval cues that are available to the subject at the time of the retention test.

Earlier it was remarked that drugs that only act outside the CNS do not produce dissociative effects in laboratory animals. The original evidence for this conclusion came from an elegant series of experiments carried out by Overton

---

statistical analyses reported by Hinrichsen and his associates; in certain critical comparisons, the degrees of freedom for the error term are twice as large as they should be. On reanalysis, the data do not appear to support unequivocally a dissociation hypothesis. The second study was performed by Peterson (1974), who has claimed to have found reliable evidence of SDR using some memory tasks but not others. To the best of my knowledge, no detailed report of this study has been published (Petersen's 1974 report consisted of a one-paragraph abstract); hence the data from the experiment are not currently available for public inspection.

(1964, 1966). Using rats as subjects, Overton was able to show that the ability of drug-state changes to produce dissociation did not appear to be based on sensory cues provided by the drugs; his efforts to mimic the effects of drug-state changes using selected interoceptive and exteroceptive cues were repeatedly unsuccessful. Several, more recent, experiments using laboratory animals lend additional support to the notion that dissociation critically depends on direct effects of a drug on the brain and not simply on the occurrence of a mélange of peripheral nervous system reactions (e.g., Downey, 1975; Overton, 1971, 1973).

The role of central vs. peripheral actions of drugs in the occurrence of dissociative effects in man is presently unclear. Most experimental studies of human SDR completed to date have involved administration of drugs in doses sufficient to produce extensive actions upon both central and peripheral nervous systems. It is interesting to note, however, that robust SDR effects have been demonstrated using a 1 mg dose of physostigmine (Weingartner, 1977), a drug known to have relatively insignificant stimulus properties (Overton, 1971). In fact, several of the subjects in the physostigmine study were unable to reliably discriminate between drug and placebo treatments when asked to do so upon completion of their participation in the experiment. Although the physostigmine results are consistent with the hypothesis that CNS-active drugs need not produce readily discriminable peripheral effects in order to promote dissociation of human retrieval, it is clear that many more experiments will need to be done before the issue of centrally vs. noncentrally mediated SDR can be definitively settled.

One final point will be made concerning drugs that produce dissociative effects in man, and this has to do with the distinction between asymmetric and symmetric SDR. Basically, asymmetric SDR refers to the finding that information "transfers" less completely in the direction of drug state to drug-free state (DN) than in the reverse direction (ND). Asymmetric SDR effects have been demonstrated using several psychoactive drugs, including alcohol (e.g., Goodwin et al., 1969), marijuana (e.g., Darley et al., 1974), and physostigmine (Weingartner, 1977). The conceptual significance of asymmetric dissociative effects is debatable. Darley et al. (1974) invoked the concept of asymmetric SDR to account for their finding that marijuana facilitated recall of words studied during a prior state of intoxication. These authors claimed that the concept afforded a "parsimonious and intuitively reasonable explanation" of their data, "particularly since drug users commonly report that events experienced while intoxicated are not remembered until the drug is ingested again at a later time [p. 148]." Arguments against the utility of the concept of asymmetric dissociation have been offered by both Overton (1972, 1974) and Deutsch and Roll (1973). Working with data collected from infrahuman subjects, these investigators have shown that asymmetric dissociation may result simply from the summation of a symmetric state-dependent effect (i.e., impaired transfer under conditions DN *and* ND) with other drug effects such as drug-induced impairment of memory consolidation or facilitation of test performance. More work is needed to determine whether the "summation" hypothesis can be extended to account for asymmetric dissociative effects seen in man. Until then the utility of the concept of asymmetric SDR will remain open to question.

Differential task "sensitivity." Many investigators have observed that SDR can be readily demonstrated in normal human adults using some memory tasks but not others. For instance, Goodwin et al. (1969) reported that serial recall of sentences of varying meaningfulness was asymmetrically state dependent for alcohol but found no evidence of dissociation using a picture-recognition task. Employing a comparable dose of alcohol, Weingartner and Faillace (1971) demonstrated symmetric SDR using a multitrial, free-recall procedure, but found no indication that reproduction of subject-generated associations to verbal stimuli was facilitated by restoration of the drug state in which the associations originally were produced. The finding that memory tasks differ with respect to their "sensitivity" as instruments for demonstrating SDR is not unique to studies involving alcohol. Darley et al. (1974), for example, used the drug state induced by oral administration of 20 mg THC to demonstrate dissociative effects on free recall – but not recognition – of common words. Differential task sensitivity also has been observed in studies using amobarbital (Ley et al., 1972), isoflurane (Adam et al., 1974), and physostigmine (Weingartner, 1977).

How do we account for the finding that some memory tasks appear more sensitive to the occurrence of dissociative effects than some others? One approach to this question is based on the idea that any given memory task can be partitioned into separately identifiable components and that the magnitude of dissociative effects may vary depending upon the extent to which these various components are present or absent in various tasks (Tulving, 1976a). Thus, for instance, Goodwin et al. (1969) suggested that a "word-association task, measuring single-trial, 'self-generated' learning, may be particularly useful in studying dissociation [p. 1359]." Actually, the evidence for this hypothesis is rather weak. Six experiments have been published that used a word-association task of the type described by Goodwin and his colleagues (Crow & Ball, 1975; Goodwin et al., 1969; Hill et al., 1973; Stillman et al., 1974; Weingartner & Faillace, 1971; Weingartner et al., 1973). Of these, three yielded reliable evidence of SDR and three did not.

A second example of analysis by task components concerns the idea that tasks requiring the processing and utilization of order information may be especially sensitive detectors of SDR (Hill et al., 1973; Stillman et al., 1974). According to this hypothesis, a change of drug state between the study and test sessions of the experiment reduces the accessibility of information specifying temporal/spatial relations among target events and thus makes it difficult, if not impossible, for the subject to remember the serial order in which the events originally transpired. Results supportive of the "order information" hypothesis can be found in a number of experimental studies. Weingartner et al. (1973), for instance, reported that alcohol facilitated serial reproduction of verbal free associations that originally had been generated during a comparable state of intoxication. Furthermore, Ley et al. (1972) found that serial recall of nonsense syllables was symmetrically state dependent for amobarbital. Additional evidence attesting to the sensitivity of tasks requiring the processing and utilization of order information can be found in papers by Goodwin et al. (1969), Hill et al. (1973), and Stillman et al. (1974). Although findings reported to date are generally consistent with predictions derived from the order-information hypothesis, it is not clear how this hypothesis could account for the extreme sensitivity of tasks involving long-term, nominally noncued *free* recall of target items, where order of item output need not — and typically does not — mimic the order in which the items were originally presented. Nine papers have been found that report the results of a total of 13 delayed free-recall "tasks"[2] (Adam et al., 1974; Bustamante et al., 1968, 1970; Darley et al., 1974; Eich et al., 1975; Jones, 1973; Weingartner, 1977; Weingartner & Faillace, 1971; Weingartner et al., 1976). Of these 13 tasks, 12 (92%) yielded evidence of SDR. This finding appears all the more remarkable in view of the fact that evidence of state-dependent free recall has been obtained using six different drugs, five different types of target items, and four different retention intervals. It is, of course, conceivable that processing and utilization of order information may be involved in delayed free-recall tasks (see Murdock, 1974), but on purely empirical grounds it would appear that accessibility of information specifying semantic or conceptual relations among to-be-remembered events is the critical determinant of free-recall performance (see, for example, Anderson & Bower, 1973; Tulving, 1968; Wallace, 1970). Still, the order-information hypothesis is ingenious, plausible, and consistent with the results of at least some studies, and it clearly merits continued experimental analysis.

Yet a third example of analysis by task components has to do with the idea that SDR effects may critically depend for their occurrence on the presence or absence of specific retrieval cues in the cognitive environment of the rememberer at the time of attempted retrieval. As the story behind this hypothesis is rather involved, the issue of "cue-specific dissociation" will be taken up separately in the next section of the paper.

---

[2] In some studies, one and the same memory task (e.g., single-trial free recall) has been used in conjunction with two or more effective drug doses (e.g., high and low concentrations of isoflurane in Adam et al., 1974) or with two or more different types of target items (e.g., high- and low-imagery words in Weingartner et al., 1976). In this paper, each unique combination of drug dose and type of target item will be regarded as a separate "task."

Cue-Specific Dissociation

We begin with the observation that utilization of stored information never occurs "spontaneously"; retrieval is always initiated by a stimulus, a query, or a cue (Tulving, 1976b). In certain tasks, such as single-trial free recall (see Tulving, 1968), retrieval appears to take place in the absence of any specific instigators; nevertheless, we assume that "invisible" cues guide the subject's retrieval efforts. In other tasks, such as paired-associate learning, retrieval appears to be effected by "intralist" cues, as when, for example, the stimulus member of a pair of associated words is provided to the subject as a cue for remembering the response member of the pair. And in tasks requiring recognition rather than reproduction of target items, information necessary for retrieval is conveyed by "copy" cues – cues nominally identical to the to-be-remembered items. In the remainder of this section we will critically examine evidence bearing on the hypothesis that tasks most sensitive to the detection of dissociative effects are those in which utilization of stored information is mediated by invisible or subject-generated retrieval cues, rather than by intralist or copy cues.

The first piece of relevant evidence comes from an experiment carried out a few years ago by this writer in collaboration with Chris Gillin, Dick Stillman, and Herb Weingartner (Eich et al., 1975). In this experiment, each of 15 college students alternately studied and was tested for retention of a long list of common words under the four experimental conditions – NN, ND, DN, and DD – where D and N represent the drug states induced by smoking a marijuana cigarette containing 10 mg and (effectively) 0 mg THC, respectively. One experimental condition was completed per day with 2 or 3 days separating successive conditions. A Latin-square design was used to determine the order in which each subject completed the four experimental conditions.

In the study phase of every experimental condition, subjects were presented a list composed of 12 taxonomic categories, each category consisting of a category name (e.g., *a flower*) and four instances of the category (e.g., *zinnia, tulip, rose, jonquil*). Participants were informed that approximately 4 hours following list presentation they would be asked to recall the 48 category instances (12 categories X 4 instances per category), but not the 12 category names. Four equivalent lists were generated, one for each experimental condition. Lists were read once at a rate of roughly 1.5 sec per category name or category instance.

In the test session of every experimental condition, subjects were administered two different tests of retention of the category instances studied earlier that day. In both tests the subjects' task was to recall as many category instances as possible in any convenient order. Furthermore, both tests required written responses and were self-paced. The critical difference between the two examinations was that in the test of *cued recall* (CR) subjects were provided with a list of the 12 category names as an aid in remembering the category instances, whereas in the test of *uncued recall* (UR) subjects were not reminded of the category names and hence were required to recall the category instances without benefit of specific, experimenter-provided cues. The CR test was always administered immediately following completion of the UR test.

The mean percentages of category instances recalled as a function of study state (N or D), test state (N or D), and test type (UR or CR) are depicted in Figure 1. Inspection of the UR data reveals that category instances studied under drug were better recalled under drug than under drug-free conditions ($p < .01$). It also can be seen that category instances studied under drug-free conditions were somewhat better remembered in the N than in the D state; however, this difference was not statistically reliable ($p > .05$). Thus, results in the UR test suggest that nominally noncued, free recall of category instances is asymmetrically state dependent for marijuana.

Results of the CR test point to an entirely different conclusion. As portrayed in Figure 1, there is no evidence of a crossover between study and test drug states with respect to cued recall of category instances and hence no indication of dissociated retrieval. Thus, results of the marijuana study suggest that:

1. The occurrence of SDR effects is limited to experimental situations where utilization of stored information critically depends on the operation of invisible or subject-generated retrieval cues.

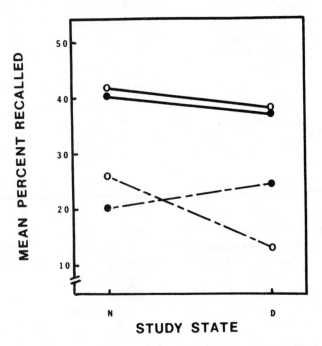

FIGURE 1   Recall of category instances (adapted from Eich et al., 1975). Key to graph: unfilled circles – test in drug-free (N) state; filled circles – test in drug (D) state; dashed lines – uncued recall; solid lines – cued recall.

2. The deleterious effect of a state change on performance in a test of nominally noncued, free recall can be completely negated by the provision of appropriate intralist cues (category names).

Additional evidence in support of the hypothesis that tasks most sensitive to the occurrence of SDR effects are those in which invisible cues guide retrieval is available in the current experimental literature. Twelve papers have been found that report the results of a total of 17 tasks involving nominally noncued, free or serial recall of target events (Adam et al., 1974; Bustamante et al., 1968, 1970; Darley et al., 1974; Eich et al., 1975; Goodwin et al., 1969; Hill et al., 1973; Jones, 1973; Stillman et al., 1974; Weingartner, 1977; Weingartner & Faillace, 1971; Weingartner et al., 1976). Of these 17 uncued-recall tasks, reliable evidence of dissociated retrieval was found in 14 (82%). This value contrasts sharply with findings derived from tasks involving cued recall of target events. Results of a total of 20 tasks pertaining either to paired-associate learning, negative transfer (viz. $A - B_r$ interference designs), prompted recall of free associations, or category cuing (as in the marijuana study described above) are available for examination (Crow & Ball, 1975; Eich et al., 1975; Goodwin et al., 1969; Hill et al., 1973; Hurst, Radlow, Chubb, & Bagley, 1969; Ley et al., 1972; Osborn et al., 1967; Parker, Birnbaum, & Noble, 1976; Rickles et al., 1973; Roffman, Marshall, Silverstein, Karkalas, Smith, & Lal, 1972; Tarter, 1970; Weingartner, 1977; Weingartner & Faillace, 1971; Weingartner et al., 1973). Only 7 of these 20 cued-recall tasks (35%) yielded reliable evidence of dissociated retrieval. Finally, 7 articles have been found that describe the results of a total of 10 tasks involving recognition of target events (Adam et al., 1974; Crow & Ball, 1975; Darley et al., 1974; Goodwin et al., 1969; Osborn et al., 1967; Parker et al., 1976; Wickelgren, 1975). Results indicative of SDR were obtained in only 2 of these 10 recognition tasks (20%).

Table 1 summarizes our discussion of the relation between task type (uncued recall, cued recall, and recognition) and task outcome with respect to the occurrence and nonoccurrence of SDR effects. Two points are worth noting about the pattern of results depicted in the table. First, human SDR clearly appears to be a cue-specific phenomenon: evidence of dissociative effects is far more likely to emerge in tasks where utilization of stored information critically depends on the operation of invisible or subject-generated retrieval cues (i.e., tasks involving uncued recall) than in tasks where retrieval is mediated either by intralist or copy cues (i.e., tasks involving either cued recall or recognition). Though it appears in Table 1 that cued-recall tasks are somewhat more sensitive to the occurrence of dissociative effects in comparison with recognition tasks — evidence of SDR was found in 35% and 20% of the cued-recall and recognition tasks, respectively — the difference between these values does not approach statistical significance ($p > .25$; difference between two proportions test). Both values, however, are significantly lower ($ps < .01$) than the score obtained for the uncued-recall tasks (82%). Second, in view of the fact that only 23 of the 47

TABLE 1
Relation Between Task Type and Task Outcome with
Respect to the Occurrence of State-Dependent Retrieval[a]

	Task outcome	
Task type	+ SDR	– SDR
Uncued recall	14	3
Cued recall	7	13
Recognition	2	8
Totals	23	24

[a]Values listed under the columns marked "+ SDR" and "– SDR" are the numbers of tasks in which reliable evidence of state-dependent retrieval (SDR) was and was not obtained, respectively. References are provided in the text.

tasks included in Table 1 yielded reliable evidence of SDR, it seems especially important to recognize that human SDR is a cue-specific phenomenon. Failure to appreciate the cue-specific nature of human SDR may lead one to incorrectly conclude, as did Hilgard and Bower (1975, p. 547), that evidence for dissociative effects in man "rests on precarious grounds."

The observation that SDR effects are not likely to obtain in tasks involving either cued recall or recognition of target events provides some insight into several puzzling findings reported in the current literature. For instance, the inability of Hurst et al. (1969) and Roffman et al. (1972) to demonstrate SDR effects in normal adults using clinical doses of amphetamine is understandable, given the fact that both teams of investigators employed paired-associate learning procedures to study dissociation. Similarly, it is not surprising that Lisman (1974) failed to demonstrate state-dependent effects in drinking alcoholics in view of the choice of his tasks (paired-associate learning and recognition). The same argument also may apply to the unsuccessful attempt of Osborn et al. (1967) to demonstrate dissociation using high doses of thiopental.

In summary, evidence gleaned from a number of experimental studies appears to justify the conclusion that human SDR is a cue-specific phenomenon; i.e., reliable evidence of dissociation is more likely to emerge in tasks where retrieval of stored information is mediated by subject-generated cues rather than by intralist or copy cues. This conclusion provides a partial explanation of why certain memory tasks differ in their sensitivity as instruments for demonstrating SDR and affords some insight into a number of other puzzling findings reported in the literature. Now that we find ourselves in possession of some rather convincing evidence that the presence or absence of specific retrieval cues plays an important role in the occurrence of dissociative effects in man, we may begin to formulate theories that speak to the cue-specific nature of human SDR. A few of the many questions that might be profitably entertained in the quest for a theoretic account of human SDR will be posed in the next and concluding section of the paper.

Prospectus

The state of the art with respect to research on human state-dependent retrieval has changed dramatically in the past 10 years. Doubts as to the reliability and robustness of SDR effects have been largely dispelled, some of the necessary conditions for demonstrating SDR in the laboratory setting have been elucidated, and a sense of the practical or applied significance of the human SDR phenomenon has slowly, perhaps inexorably, evolved.

Where will research on dissociative effects in man lead from here? It is not possible at this time to state with precision what the important issues for future research will be. However, several questions do appear central in understanding the human SDR phenomenon and will likely be the foci of empirical and theoretic interest in the years ahead. For instance, is conscious awareness of a change of drug state between the study and test sessions of the experiment a necessary condition for demonstrating SDR? Will retrieval fail if the study and test sessions take place in the context of different doses of the same drug (Jones, 1974)? Why should tasks involving uncued recall of to-be-remembered events appear more sensitive to the occurrence of dissociative effects in comparison with tasks involving either cued recall or recognition? How is it possible that appropriate intralist retrieval cues (viz., category names) completely negate the deleterious effect of a state change on uncued recall of category instances, when surely it is the case that cuing per se does not serve to reintroduce the original drug state (Roediger, 1975)? Can the amnesic effect of a state change be attenuated by the provision of specific *extralist* retrieval cues — cues not present at the time of initial encoding of target events? Is there a fundamental difference between dissociative effects associated with disturbance of affect or mood and those produced by drugs, or do pharmacologic and nonpharmacologic manifestations of SDR differ solely at the level of empirical operations?

Questions regarding the applicability of SDR research findings to a variety of "real-life" behavioral problems and phenomena are also likely to come under close inspection in the coming years. What, for instance, is the nature of the relation between SDR and drug abuse (see Overton, 1973)? It is conceivable that SDR may be produced by drug effects that are also reinforcing; hence, SDR and drug abuse may be correlated but not causally related phenomena (Harris & Balster, 1970; Overton, 1972, 1973). On the other hand, memory for the dysphoric side effects of drug intoxication may be irrecoverable in the drug-free state; hence, SDR may be a causal factor in drug abuse. Some evidence in support of a causal relation between SDR and drug abuse has been reported by Tamerin, Weiner, Poppen, Steinglass, and Mendelson (1971), who found that alcoholics tend to selectively forget unpleasant experiences that occurred during a state of alcohol intoxication (see Overton, 1973).

Drug abuse is not the only practical problem that may be relevant to notions of human dissociated retrieval. Several theorists (e.g., Kamano, 1966) have conjectured that psychotherapy, when conducted in the course of ongoing chemotherapy, may lead to insights or coping strategies that are state specific. Gains made in the course of psychotherapy may be lost when the drug regimen is discontinued. This line of thought also is reflected in Storm and Smart's (1965) suggestion that alcoholics may benefit more from either operant or dynamically oriented treatment programs when the patients are intoxicated during therapy.

State-dependent retrieval may also have important implications in the analysis of "flashback" phenomena associated with LSD use (Fischer & Landon, 1972), in understanding some of the problems involved in sticking to a medication schedule (cf. Hare & Willcox, 1967), in the diagnosis and treatment of hyperactivity in children (Swanson & Kinsbourne, 1976), and in explanations of why some surgical and dental patients show postoperative amnesia for events that occurred in the context of anesthetic analgesia — unless recall is attempted in a comparable anesthetic state or under hypnosis (Cheek, 1962; Levinson, 1965; Overton, 1968).

Clearly, students of human state dependence have shown considerable ingenuity in attempting to apply data and theory generated within the laboratory to problems and phenomena encountered outside the laboratory. This approach seems desirable for several reasons, not the least important of which is the tendency of funding agencies to look favorably upon research that has applied as well as theoretic significance. Of course, all the potential applications mentioned above must at present be regarded simply as speculative albeit interesting ideas. But there appears no compelling reason why these potential applications cannot be converted into accomplished facts in the years to come.

ACKNOWLEDGMENTS

Preparation of this chapter was facilitated by the support of the Laboratory of Clinical Science, Section on Clinical Neuropharmacology, National Institute of Mental Health, Bethesda, Maryland. Gus Craik, Patt McCauley, Norm Park, Dan Schacter, Dick Stillman, Norm Slamecka, Endel Tulving, Mike Watkins, and Herb Weingartner provided thoughtful criticisms of the evolving manuscript.

REFERENCES

Adam, N., Castro, A. D., & Clark, D. L. State-dependent learning with a general anesthetic (Isoflurane) in man. *T. –I. –T. Journal of Life Sciences,* 1974, *4,* 125–134.
Anderson, J. R., & Bower, G. H. *Human associative memory.* Washington, D. C.: Winston & Sons, 1973.

Berger, B. D., & Stein, L. An analysis of the learning deficits produced by scopolamine. *Psychopharmacologia*, 1969, *14*, 271–283.

Bower, G. H. A selective review of organizational factors in memory. In E. Tulving & W. Donaldson (Eds.), *Organization of memory*. New York: Academic Press, 1972.

Bustamante, J. A., Jordán, A., Vila, M., González, A., & Insua, A. State dependent learning in humans. *Physiology & Behavior*, 1970, *5*, 793–796.

Bustamante, J. A., Rosselló, A., Jordán, A., Pradere, E., & Insua, A. Learning and drugs. *Physiology & Behavior*, 1968, *3*, 553–555.

Cheek, D. B. Importance of recognizing that surgical patients behave as though hypnotized. *American Journal of Clinical Hypnosis*, 1962, *4*, 227–236.

Crosland, H. R. A qualitative analysis of the process of forgetting. *Psychological Monographs*, 1921, *29*, (No. 130).

Crow, L. T., & Ball, C. Alcohol state-dependency and autonomic reactivity. *Psychophysiology*, 1975, *12*, 702–706.

Darley, C. F., Tinklenberg, J. R., Roth, W. T., & Atkinson, R. C. The nature of storage deficits and state-dependent retrieval under marihuana. *Psychopharmacologia*, 1974, *37*, 139–149.

Deutsch, J. A., & Roll, S. K. Alcohol and asymmetrical state-dependency: a possible explanation. *Behavioral Biology*, 1973, *8*, 273–278.

Downey, D. J. State-dependent learning with centrally and noncentrally active drugs. *Bulletin of the Psychonomic Society*, 1975, *5*, 281–284.

Eich, J. E., Weingartner, H., Stillman, R. C., & Gillin, J. C. State-dependent accessibility of retrieval cues in the retention of a categorized list. *Journal of Verbal Learning and Verbal Behavior*, 1975, *14*, 408–417.

Fischer, R., & Landon, G. M. On the arousal state-dependent recall of "subconscious" experience: state-boundness. *British Journal of Psychiatry*, 1972, *120*, 159–172.

Goodwin, D. W. Blackouts and alcohol induced memory dysfunction. In N. K. Mello & J. H. Mendelson (Eds.), *Recent advances in studies of alcoholism*. Rockville, Md.: National Institute of Mental Health, 1971.

Goodwin, D. W., Powell, B., Bremer, D., Hoine, H., & Stern, J. Alcohol and recall: State dependent effects in man. *Science*, 1969, *163*, 1358–1360.

Hare, E. H., & Willcox, D. R. Do psychiatric in-patients take their pills? *British Journal of Psychiatry*, 1967, *113*, 1435–1437.

Harris, R. T., & Balster, R. L. An analysis of psychological dependence. In R. T. Harris, W. H. McIsaac, & C. R. Schuster, Jr. (Eds.), *Advances in mental science II: Drug dependence*. Austin: University of Texas Press, 1970.

Hilgard, E. R., & Bower, G. H. *Theories of learning* (4th ed.). Englewood Cliffs, N. J.: Prentice-Hall, 1975.

Hill, S. Y., Schwin, R., Powell, B., & Goodwin, D. W. State-dependent effects of marihuana on human memory. *Nature*, 1973, *243*, 241–242.

Hinrichsen, J. J., Katahn, M., & Levenson, R. W. Alcohol-induced state-dependent learning in non-alcoholics. *Pharmacology, Biochemistry & Behavior*, 1974, *2*, 293–296.

Hollingworth, H. L. *Psychology: Its facts and principles*. New York: Appleton, 1928.

Hurst, P. M., Radlow, R., Chubb, N. C., & Bagley, S. K. Effects of d-amphetamine on acquisition, persistence, and recall. *American Journal of Psychology*, 1969, *82*, 307–319.

Jones, B. M. Memory impairment on the ascending and descending limbs of the blood alcohol curve. *Journal of Abnormal Psychology*, 1973, *82*, 24–32.

Jones, B. M. Circadian variation in the effects of alcohol on cognitive performance. *Quarterly Journal of Studies on Alcohol*, 1974, *35*, 1212–1219.

Kamano, D. K. Selective review of effects of discontinuation of drug treatment: Some implications and problems. *Psychological Reports*, 1966, *19*, 743–749.

Levinson, B. W. States of awareness during general anaesthesia. *British Journal of Anaesthesia*, 1965, *37*, 544–546.

Lewin, K. *A dynamic theory of personality*. New York: McGraw-Hill, 1935.

Ley, P., Jain, V. K., Swinson, R. P., Eaves, D., Bradshaw, P. W., Kincey, J. A., Crowder, R., & Abbiss, S. A state-dependent learning effect produced by amylobarbitone sodium. *British Journal of Psychiatry*, 1972, *120*, 511–515.

Light, L. L., & Carter–Sobell, L. Effects of changed semantic context on recognition memory. *Journal of Verbal Learning and Verbal Behavior*, 1970, *9*, 1–11.

Lisman, S. A. Alcoholic "blackout": State dependent learning? *Archives of General Psychiatry*, 1974, *30*, 46–53.

McGeoch, J. A. A bibliography of human learning. *Psychological Bulletin*, 1933, *30*, 1–62.

McGeoch, J. A. Learning. In E. G. Boring, H. S. Langfeld, & H. P. Weld (Eds.), *Introduction to psychology*. New York: Wiley, 1939.

Melton, A. W. Implications of short-term memory for a general theory of memory. *Journal of Verbal Learning and Verbal Behavior*, 1963, *2*, 1–21.

Murdock, B. B., Jr. *Human memory: Theory and data*. Potomac, Md.: Lawrence Erlbaum Associates, 1974.

Osborn, A. G., Bunker, J. P., Cooper, L. F., Frank, G. S., & Hilgard, E. R. Effects of thiopental sedation on learning and memory. *Science*, 1967, *157*, 574–576.

Overton, D. A. State-dependent or "dissociated" learning produced with pentobarbital. *Journal of Comparative and Physiological Psychology*, 1964, *57*, 3–12.

Overton, D. A. State-dependent learning produced by depressants and atropine-like drugs. *Psychopharmacologia*, 1966, *10*, 6–31.

Overton, D. A. Dissociated learning in drug states (state-dependent learning). In D. H. Efron, J. O. Cole, J. Levine, & R. Wittenborn (Eds.), *Psychopharmacology: A review of progress, 1957–1967*. Washington, D. C.: U. S. Government Printing Office, 1968.

Overton, D. A. Discriminative control of behavior by drug states. In T. Thompson & R. Pickens (Eds.), *Stimulus properties of drugs*. New York: Appleton-Century-Crofts, 1971.

Overton, D. A. State-dependent learning produced by alcohol and its relevance to alcoholism. In B. Kissen & H. Begleiter (Eds.), *The biology of alcoholism: Vol. II: Physiology and behavior*. New York: Plenum Press, 1972.

Overton, D. A. State-dependent learning produced by addicting drugs. In S. Fisher & A. M. Freedman (Eds.), *Opiate addiction: Origins and treatment*. Washington, D. C.: Winston & Sons, 1973.

Overton, D. A. Experimental methods for the study of state-dependent learning. *Federation Proceedings*, 1974, *33*, 1800–1813.

Parker, E. S., Birnbaum, I. M., & Noble, E. P. Alcohol and memory: Storage and state dependency. *Journal of Verbal Learning and Verbal Behavior*, 1976, *15*, 691–702.

Pear, T. H. *Remembering and forgetting*. New York: Dutton, 1922.

Petersen, R. C. Evidence for alcohol state-dependent learning in man. *Federation Proceedings*, 1974, *33*, 550.

Reiff, R., & Scheerer, M. *Memory and hypnotic age regression*. New York: International Universities Press, Inc., 1959.

Rickles, W. H., Jr., Cohen, M. J., Whitaker, C. A., & McIntyre, K. E. Marihuana induced state-dependent verbal learning. *Psychopharmacologia*, 1973, *30*, 349–354.

Roediger, H. L. Current status of research on retrieval processes in memory. *Polygraph*, 1975, *4*, 304–310.

Roffman, M., Marshall, P., Silverstein, A., Karkalas, J., Smith, N., & Lal, H. Failure to demonstrate "amphetamine state" controlling learned behavior in humans. In J. M. Singh, L. Miller, & H. Lal (Eds.), *Drug addiction. Vol. 2: Clinical and socio-legal aspects*. Mt. Kisco, N.Y.: Futura Publishing Co., 1972.

Semon, R. *Die Mneme* (1904). English translation by L. Simon. London: George Allen & Unwin, Ltd., 1921.

Stillman, R. C., Weingartner, H., Wyatt, R. J., Gillin, J. C., & Eich, J. E. State-dependent (dissociative) effects of marihuana on human memory. *Archives of General Psychiatry,* 1974, *31,* 81–85.

Storm, T., & Smart, R. G. Dissociation: A possible explanation of some features of alcoholism, and implications for treatment. *Quarterly Journal of Studies on Alcohol,* 1965, *26,* 111–115.

Swanson, J. M., & Kinsbourne, M. Stimulant-related state-dependent learning in hyperactive children. *Science,* 1976, *192,* 1354–1357.

Tamerin, J. S., Weiner, S., Poppen, R., Steinglass, P., & Mendelson, J. H. Alcohol and memory: Amnesia and short-term memory function during experimentally induced intoxication. *American Journal of Psychiatry,* 1971, *127,* 1659–1664.

Tarter, R. E. Dissociate effects of ethyl alcohol. *Psychonomic Science,* 1970, *20,* 342–343.

Tulving, E. Theoretical issues in free recall. In T. R. Dixon & D. L. Horton (Eds.), *Verbal behavior and general behavior theory.* Englewood Cliffs, N. J.: Prentice-Hall, 1968.

Tulving, E. Episodic and semantic memory. In E. Tulving & W. Donaldson (Eds.), *Organization of memory.* New York: Academic Press, 1972.

Tulving, E. Paper presented at the Conference on Alcohol and Memory, Laguna Beach, Calif., September 1976. (a)

Tulving, E. Rôle de la mémoire sémantique dans le stockage et la récupération de l'information épisodique. In S. Ehrlich & E. Tulving (Eds.), *La mémoire sémantique.* Paris: Bulletin de Psychologie, 1976. (b)

Wallace, W. P. Consistency of emission order in free recall. *Journal of Verbal Learning and Verbal Behavior,* 1970, *9,* 58–68.

Weingartner, H. Human state-dependent learning. In B. T. Ho, D. Richards, III, & D. L. Shute (Eds.), *Drug discrimination and state-dependent learning.* New York: Academic Press, 1977 (in press).

Weingartner, H., Adefris, W., Eich, J. E., & Murphy, D. L. Encoding-imagery specificity in alcohol state-dependent learning. *Journal of Experimental Psychology: Human Learning and Memory,* 1976, *2,* 83–87.

Weingartner, H., Eich, J. E., & Allen, R. Alcohol state-dependent associative processes. *Proceedings of the American Psychological Association,* 1973, *8,* 1009–1010.

Weingartner, H., & Faillace, L. A. Alcohol state-dependent learning in man. *Journal of Nervous and Mental Disease,* 1971, *153,* 395–406.

Wickelgren, W. A. Alcoholic intoxication and memory storage dynamics. *Memory & Cognition,* 1975, *3,* 385–389.

11
State-Dependent Storage and Retrieval of Experience While Intoxicated

Herbert Weingartner

Laboratory of Psychology and Psychopathology
National Institute of Mental Health

Dennis L. Murphy

Clinical Neuropharmacology Branch
National Institute of Mental Health

The brain is sensitive to the effects of depressant drugs such as alcohol in terms of its neurophysiological and neurochemical responsiveness and consequent changes in behavior. Each of these systems of measuring the response to alcohol intoxication is pertinent to understanding the biological—behavioral effects of alcohol, including its reinforcing and addictive properties. This paper focuses on some specific cognitive and behavioral effects of alcohol and what these tell us about both the action of this drug on the central nervous system and its role in altering cognitive processes. Such investigations may also provide a convenient tool for studying some of the biological determinants of normal information processing, storage, and retrieval as these are reflected in an examination of how events are processed, recorded, and recovered under specifiable altered brain-state conditions. Thus, investigations of the alcohol response provide an opportunity to integrate cognitive findings generated from clinical, psychopharmacological, and human information processing approaches to the study of higher cortical functions in man.

In this report we present three studies that highlight some of the qualitative and quantitative changes in thinking and memory as these occur in the intoxicated state. These findings serve the purpose of illustrating how current models of information processing can be used to further understand the psychology of the intoxicated state, factors that might relate to the reinforcing properties of alcohol, and cognitive factors associated with long-term effects of alcohol in the alcohol abuser. The findings are also a pertinent testing ground for some of the issues thought to be particularly germane in accounting for information storage, memory retrieval, and the relationships between the storage-retrieval environment in ultimately determining whether previous experience can be remembered under specific retrieval conditions. Some of the salient features of current models of memory storage and retrieval that have been used to reflect aspects of cognition in the intoxicated state also represent the foci of current theories of information processing in man. These include:

1. Notions of memory storage stages such as versions of short- vs. long-term memory store (Wickelgren, 1973) as contrasted with concepts of depth or elaborateness of information processing (Craik & Lockhart, 1972).

2. Contextualism as it determines the specific processing and encoding of input and the necessary conditions that would prevail for the successful retrieval of some episodic event (Tulving & Thomson, 1973).

3. Measurement and definition of structures previously learned and stored in memory, their role in transforming experienced events, and their unique relevance in accounting for the encoding of events in the altered brain state (Weingartner, Snyder, Faillace, & Marley, 1970).

4. The role of brain state-specific accessing strategies that account for how past events are retrieved from memory (Weingartner & Murphy, 1977).

The studies summarized here contribute data that reflect on each of these systems of variables as descriptors of cognition in the intoxicated vs. sober state. These findings also provide some convergent support for some of the current theories of memory that posit an intimate interrelationship between events and context that define storage and retrieval of experience.

Not all facets of experience appear to be altered or disrupted in the intoxicated state. Task- and stimulus-specific responses to alcohol suggest that impairment in higher cortical functions is generally related to task complexity and that the subtler, less salient, or less easily encoded events are more susceptible to change and disruption when processed in the alcohol-intoxicated state. Some of the findings presented below are pertinent to this issue. Other findings presented here, as well as those described elsewhere, seem to indicate that the immediate recall of experienced events is less disrupted than subsequent delayed retrieval of those events, particularly when the opportunity to rehearse or recapitulate events is prevented. Such effects suggest that in the intoxicated state the formation of some permanent trace of experience or its consolidation is somehow disrupted. This characteristic of the alcohol response shares some features in common with memory changes associated with hippocampal-temporal-amygdala brain lesions in man (Milner, 1970) and postlearning-specific and nonspecific brain state arousal effects on previously learned responses in animals (McGaugh & Herz, 1972) as well as in man (Weingartner, Hall, Murphy, & Weinstein, 1976).

Processing, storage, and retrieval of experience while intoxicated is not simply disrupted; there also appear to be changes in how events are interpreted, encoded, and transformed in this altered brain state. That is, the strategies used to interpret and store experience are somehow different when intoxicated compared to the strategies used while in a sober state. This change in the interpretation of events appears to play a major role in the induction of dissociative or state-dependent learning and memory retrieval that occurs in the intoxicated state (Goodwin, Powell, Bremer, Hoine, & Stern, 1969; Weingartner & Faillace, 1971). Such dissociations are manifest when experiences stored while intoxicated are more completely recalled in a later, comparable state of intoxication than in the albeit cognitively "more effective" sober state. State-dependent learning and state-dependent retrieval, as seen in the alcohol-intoxicated state, appear to have important implications for understanding some of the unique characteristics that define the intoxicated state. The dissociative phenomenon also lends strong support to theories of information processing that emphasize the interdependence of the storage and retrieval context in defining what has been learned. The findings presented here suggest that brain state seems to serve as a kind of context at the time of storage and retrieval in much the same manner as an informational context serves to determine the unique encoding of an event and the retrieval conditions necessary for its recall (Tulving & Thomson, 1973).

EXPERIMENT 1

This study was designed to contrast some of the features of storage-memory decay of verbal information in the intoxicated vs. sober state. We used a free-recall measure as an estimate of how much information might be in memory store at various points in time after storage had taken place while either sober or intoxicated. The study was also designed to contrast recall of unrelated random words with subject-generated, meaningful mnemonic verbal labels that were used to identify clusters of random word-events.

Twelve male subjects (age range 21 to 26) were each run twice under sober conditions and twice intoxicated, after consuming a "cocktail" made up of 3.5 ounces, 190-proof alcohol mixed in 4 ounces of orange juice. This amount of alcohol produced a mean blood alcohol level of .10% as measured by Breathalyzer readings obtained from these subjects and measured 25 minutes after consuming the mixture. This was also the time when subjects listened to equivalent sets of random, high-frequency words (Thorndike-Lorge, 1944, A or AA words) presented auditorily at a 2-second rate. These words were then immediately recalled and recalled again 20 minutes later.

Subjects were first presented with 8 random, high-frequency common nouns. They were then required to produce a single word label that might best represent or code each of these random word-clusters. The only restrictions on the nature of the self-generated labeling response words were that they had to be single words other than members of the immediately preceding word set and not from a preceding word set. Following this, subjects were required to recall the random words. Subjects then heard the next 8-word set, which was again labeled and immediately recalled. The procedure was repeated, using 8 sets of 8 words each, 64 words in all. After the last recall attempt, subjects were engaged in a distracting activity designed to prevent rehearsal. Twenty minutes later, subjects were again asked to first recall the word labels used to identify the sets of 8 random words and then attempt recall of the 64 random word-stimuli. All subjects were first practiced with similar materials. In each condition subjects were presented with equivalent sets of words (with respect to word frequency). Sequencing of experimental conditions was systematically randomized across subjects. Only one experimental condition was run on any given day, and subjects were always run individually.

Subjects consistently reported experiencing a moderately high level of subjective intoxication, including some motor impairment and the experience of feeling high; most also experienced a dysphoric mood after consuming alcohol. Neither immediate recall of random word-sets nor the strategies by which subjects emitted responses (e.g., serial position effects) was altered or disrupted in the intoxicated state. On the other hand, the subsequent delayed recall of these same stimuli 20 minutes later was dramatically impaired when storage and retrieval occurred under intoxicated conditions as compared to the sober storage and recall state ($F = 9.4$; $df = 1, 22$; $p < .01$). This finding is described in Figure 1. The sharp decrease in free recall of random words under alcohol conditions, however, was not reflected in the delayed recall of self-generated sets of labels identifying sublists of words.

These data are consistent with a number of similar findings where recall following a time delay — while intoxicated — seems to be particularly impaired, whereas immediate recall remains relatively unaltered in the intoxicated state. It is also clear that alcoholic subjects show this same pattern of storage-retrieval changes both when intoxicated and when sober, even months following abstinence from alcohol (Weingartner & Faillace, 1971). In many ways these findings also mimic in minature what has been classically and dramatically demonstrated in patients with Korsakoff's psychosis, namely, that immediate memory is left relatively unimpaired, but the same information appears to be inaccessible after even short delay periods. Apparently, the Korsakoff subject appears to encode events inadequately at the time of information storage, and this may account for some of the recall failure following delay (Cermak, Butters, & Gerrein, 1973). These findings also share much in common with the stimulus-specific features of the memory disturbances associated with the processing of language information in dominant temporal lobe-hippocampal lesions in man (Milner, 1970; Weingartner, 1968). Perhaps a failure to encode events deeply or elaborately while intoxicated may account for some of the recall failures evidenced when events

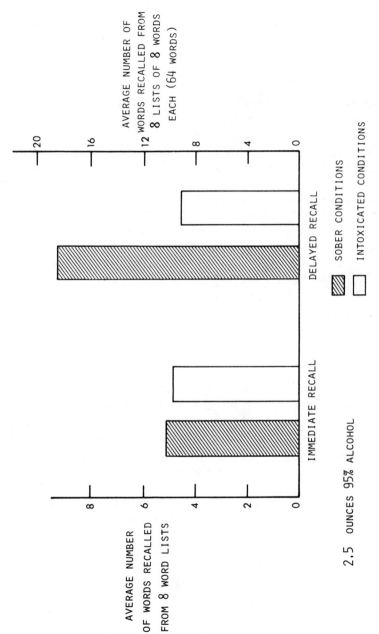

FIGURE 1 Recall of words under sober and alcohol intoxicated conditions.

are processed while subject is intoxicated. If events processed and stored while intoxicated result in the establishment of a relatively weak trace event, then this may result in more rapid trace decay or may make such a trace more suceptible to postlearning interference. It is also possible that alcohol interferes with retrieval processes so that stored events cannot be effectively accessed at the time of recall. These possibilities can be tested with currently available experimental methods.

A parallel biological view of the disruption of information processing in the intoxicated state is one that focuses on alterations of brain state arousal and its effects on memory consolidation. Operationalizing consolidation appears to be even more difficult than defining concepts such as encoding. Nonetheless, pursuing the consolidation–disruption hypothesis in accounting for impaired learning-memory in the intoxicated state may prove to be quite productive. One possible approach would be to consider the intoxicated, as compared to the sober brain state, in terms of specific and nonspecific arousal factors (Weingartner & Murphy, 1977). Alcohol, in depressing brain function, might then be studied as a change in arousal state that would then inhibit the formation of a memory trace; whereas brain state arousal, particularly postlearning, would be important in the establishment of a relatively permanent trace event (Weingartner, Hall, Murphy, & Weinstein, 1976).

EXPERIMENT 2

A number of studies have demonstrated that alcohol produces a memory dissociation so that learning that takes place while in an intoxicated state is far less effectively retrieved in the sober state than when memory storage is later searched in a similar state of intoxication. These studies usually have been accomplished in the normal subject where learning and later recall are attempted and contrasted under at least four different conditions; learn while sober–recall in a sober state; learn sober–recall while intoxicated; learn while intoxicated–recall while intoxicated; and learn intoxicated–recall sober. This design has some limitations for unequivocally uncovering dissociative effects, but nonetheless alcohol state-dependent learning can be reliably induced under certain specifiable conditions. These conditions have provided some of the findings on which are based concepts that would define some of the structure and mechanisms to account for alcohol state-dependent learning or storage (SDS) and state-dependent retrieval (SDR). For example, it has been shown that SDS–SDR is potentiated in the alcoholic subject (Weingartner & Faillace, 1971), and this effect may contribute to the alcohol blackout often reported and observed in the drinking alcoholic (Goodwin, 1971). It also appears likely that SDS–SDR is evident where time-tagged events are retrieved from memory in some orderly sequence (Eich & Weingartner, in preparation). In addition, it appears that it is possible to erase SDS–SDR by providing subjects with powerful retrieval cues at the time of recall (Eich, Weingartner, Stillman, & Gillin, 1975). It may also be necessary for subjects to subjectively experience a change in state if a memory dissociation is to appear in the disparate state (Weingartner & Murphy, 1977; Eich & Weingartner, in preparation). Finally, repeating events at the time of storage, thereby encoding them more effectively, prevents state-disparate dissociations of memory (Eich, Stillman, & Weingartner, in preparation).

One way of conceptualizing alcohol SDS–SDR is to consider it as an example of context-specific information storage and retrieval. That is, just as an informational context may induce a specific encoding strategy for storing events and therefore determine an optimal retrieval context for recall, so also might the alcohol-intoxicated state provide a stimulus context – an altered brain state – for the unique processing of experience. Similarly, as an information retrieval context may facilitate or inhibit recall as a function of the similarity of retrieval and storage context, so too might the alcohol-intoxicated brain provide a unique pharmacologically induced, neurochemical–neurophysiological context for searching memory for previously stored events. This context determines how events are interpreted and "laid down" in memory and consequently the optimal search strategy that must either be provided or self-generated in order to find previously stored events.

Since alcohol induces memory dissociations, one might expect that this drug should necessarily induce changes in the strategies used to encode or interpret ongoing events that are processed and stored in memory. Two studies that we have completed would tend to bear this out. The demonstrations are, however, weak, in part because it is quite difficult to directly measure encoding and retrieval strategies.

In one study, we examined the verbal free associations of alcoholic and control subjects while sober on one occasion and while intoxicated on another. We produced an intoxicated state as in Experiment 1. To study word encoding we used the following rationale and method. The kinds of words that freely come to mind as associations in thinking about stimuli might be expected to change in the intoxicated compared to sober state. Such changes in verbal free associates need not be thought of as mediating changes in cognition but could, nonetheless, reflect underlying alterations in the interpretation of ongoing events. In arguing such a position it is not necessary to posit a classic associational view of cognitive process but rather that associational changes do seem to reflect changes in thinking in many drug-altered brain states. (Weingartner, Snyder, Faillace, & Marley, 1970).

We used Palermo and Jenkins' noun stimuli (1964) as events to be "interpreted" by two groups of subjects – normal controls and chronic alcoholics. The subjects were tested sober on one occasion and at another time while intoxicated. Subjects were merely asked to produce a single free association to each of 20 noun stimuli in a manner similar to that used in generating the word-association norms. What we noted was that in the sober state, both alcoholic and control subjects tended to give high-frequency, commonly elicited responses to these same stimuli. Sixty percent of normal control responses had occurrence frequencies of over 50 per 500 as found in the Palermo—Jenkins norms (s.e. ± .08), whereas alcoholic subjects produced slightly fewer common responses (51% ± .13). The two groups of subjects were seen as essentially replicating the normative associations described by Palermo and Jenkins. However, when intoxicated, both groups of subjects produced a far greater number of rarer, more idiosyncratic associations, and this was particularly noticeable in the alcoholic subjects. For example, alcoholic subjects produced far fewer common responses, 20% less than were elicited in a sober state. Incidentally, it is the alcoholic subject who demonstrates a more substantial memory dissociation when compared to normal controls using the same alcohol dose (Weingartner & Faillace, 1971).

Evidence to suggest that these associational changes were not merely the product of a relaxed task-production criterion in the intoxicated state was seen when some of our subjects (10 in each group) also attempted to reproduce their free associations 20 minutes after generating them. When sober, both groups were able to reliably reproduce associations (a mean of 86%, s.e. 7%, for controls; a mean of 79%, s.e. 13%, in the alcoholic subjects). Although reproducibility of associations does decrease to 68% (s.e. 14%) in alcoholic subjects while intoxicated (it is virtually unchanged in the intoxicated normal control), it nevertheless remains quite high and does not account for the marked shift toward the production of unusual associations that characterizes the intoxicated state of the alcoholic. The basic thrust of these data are that when intoxicated, different words come to mind in processing stimuli as compared to what is generated as an appropriate associative idea or word in the sober state. Presumably this does suggest something about the fact that encoding of events is different in the sober compared to the intoxicated state.

In the next study, we again used the same amounts of alcohol mixed in juice to induce a state of intoxication in a group of young normal males (N = 12). Breathalyzer readings were obtained 25 minutes after they drank the cocktail. We studied subjects in four different conditions as in a 2 X 2 SDL design. Subjects were asked to first generate and later recall, 4 hours later, large sets (20) of self-generated sequences of associations that they produced in response to word stimuli. Recall of these associative strings was accomplished on different occasions in either a congruent or disparate state with respect to sobriety and intoxication.

We asked our subjects to generate 20 discrete free associations in response to noun stimuli chosen from the Palermo and Jenkins associative norms (1964). These stimuli had the characteristic of eliciting relatively flat response distributions, such as the word "music," which does not elicit one single response that accounts for a majority of normative subject responses. Subjects were required to generate responses as single units and not phrases and to later remember these words in the same order in which they were generated. They were always first rehearsed on this task so that they could produce all of their responses rapidly, within 3 minutes. Later, in either a congruent or disparate sober or intoxicated state, subjects were required to reproduce these associations in the same order as they initially were generated. We considered the 20 sequentially produced responses as a series of stimulus—response pairs, where each preceding response would serve as a stimulus for a subsequent response. At the time of serial recall, one response presumably would bring to mind a succeeding word, within a state-specific context. If time-tagged sequential information is inaccessible in the disparate retrieval state, then reproducing sequences of self-generated responses should reflect this deficiency.

We found that total word recall was not markedly altered when tested in these four experimental conditions. However, the same sequential pairings of words were more effectively maintained when retrieval took place in the congruent rather than in the disparate state. In other words, subjects reliably recalled items in the same sequence in congruent-state retrieval; this was less evident under disparate-state retrieval conditions. The disruption in recall of sequential information in the disparate retrieval state was reflected in the total displacement of a recalled response in the reproduced list compared to its originally generated output serial position ($F = 5.1, df = 3, 37, p < .01$).

EXPERIMENT 3

This study was designed to again test for alcohol state-dependent learning but with a focus on whether saliently or powerfully encoded stimuli would be less susceptible to dissociation in recall than less easily encoded events (Weingartner, Adefris, Eich, & Murphy, 1976). Variations in encoding were manipulated by altering characteristics of to-be-remembered events (words), rather than through the use of different orienting tasks. As in Experiment 2 we had 11 subjects learn, immediately recall, and again later recall words under 2 congruent and 2 disparate recall conditions with respect to alcohol intoxication and sobriety.

The stimuli presented for free recall, which was tested 4 hours later, were all highly common random words — a total of 20 in all, read to subjects at the rate of 1 word every 5 seconds. Ten of the words in each list were highly imageable (Paivio, Yuille, & Madigan, 1968; imagery ratings with a mean of 6.2), whereas the remaining 10 words were difficult to image (imagery ratings with a mean of 2.8). Four equivalent 20-word lists were constructed so that high- and low-imagery words were systematically randomized within each list. That is, high- and low-imagery words were distributed across all input serial positions. Different lists were presented to subjects on four different occasions, each representing one element in a 2 × 2 SDL design.

We noted a small reduction in the immediate recall of words when learning or storage took place while intoxicated ($F = 8.47$; $df = 1, 10$; $p < .01$). This recall deficit was most evident for those words that appeared in the middle of the presented lists ($F = 6.9$; $df = 4, 40$; $p < .01$). These data are displayed in Figures 2 and 3.

When recall, 4 hours later, took place in the disparate state, fewer previously recalled words were correctly recalled than under congruent storage-retrieval conditions ($F = 4.23$; $df = 3, 10$; $p < .05$). This SDS–SDR finding was not associated with any obvious changes in the manner in which subjects retrieved events from memory (e.g., immediate recall output serial position did not systematically influence recall probability). However, what was most striking was that the high-imagery words — presumably more easily or saliently encoded words — produced relatively small memory dissociation in disparate-state retrieval; whereas low-imagery words, which perhaps establish a more fragile memory trace, accounted for more of the observed alcohol-induced memory dissociations ($F = 4.3$; $df = 3, 30$; $p < .05$ for the interaction of Condition × Imagery).

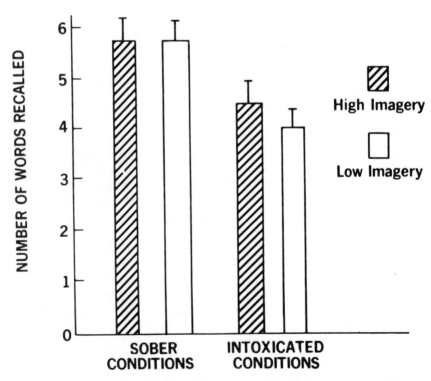

FIGURE 2   Immediate recall of words in a sober and alcohol intoxicated condition.

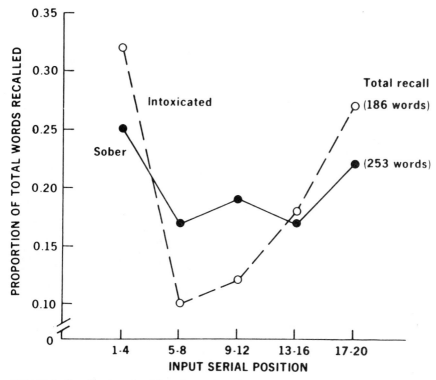

FIGURE 3   Recall of words while sober or intoxicated in relation to input serial position. (From Weingartner, Adefris, Eich, & Murphy, 1976, Fig. 1. Copyright 1976 by the American Psychological Association. Reprinted by permission.)

This last finding illustrates that memory dissociations associated with the intoxicated state can be modified not only by the manner in which retrieval is tested, e.g., free vs. cued recall (Eich, Weingartner, Stillman, & Gillin, 1975), but also by the nature of the stimuli stored in memory. Perhaps the critical issue that distinguishes dissociations seen more with low-imagery than high-imagery words is the process of imaging itself and its relevance to right- vs. left-sided cortical functioning. Might alcohol be particularly disruptive to dominant hemisphere functions that presumably are particularly involved in language processing, whereas nondominant hemisphere processing of pattern information is less sensitive to disruption in the intoxicated state? A simpler, and perhaps more attractive, notion might be that highly or easily encoded events, if represented in the brain after being consolidated (whatever that implies), are laid down in a more salient form with a representation in the brain that contains features that are hard to miss when retrieving events from memory. The subtle event, on the

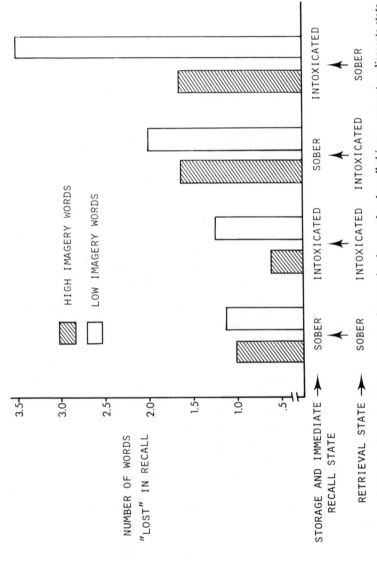

FIGURE 4 Words not retrieved from memory but previously stored and recalled in a congruent or disparate state. (From Weingartner et al., 1976, Fig. 2. Copyright 1976 by the American Psychological Association. Reprinted by permission.)

other hand, is represented by "softer," less distinctive, features that may be more easily missed, especially when some disparate-state retrieval strategy is used to search memory.

SOME CONCLUDING COMMENTS

Alcohol produces some interesting and dramatic effects on the brain. It alters the manner in which we process, store, and retrieve experience. We have at our disposal some powerful new techniques for following and describing how experiences are ordinarily dealt with in attention, perception, and memory; clearly these models have begun to be usefully applied to the study of the alcohol-intoxicated state. To date, these models have just begun to provide a picture contrasting mechanisms of information processing in the sober compared to the intoxicated state. They have barely been applied to the study of the alcohol abuser or to the long-term effects of alcohol on the brain. It would appear that research that deliberately attempts to bridge pharmacological, neurochemical, neurophysiological, clinical, and experimental psychological systems should provide a particularly productive arena for further research.

There now exist many, often conflicting, models of information processing. All of them are far from complete. The alcohol-intoxicated state can itself be used as a pharmacological tool with which to contrast and clarify the features of these different information-processing schemes. For example, it would seem that some of the clearest evidence in support of notions of encoding and retrieval specificity comes not from manipulations of informational fields at the time of storage and retrieval but from alterations of brain state at these two points in time. The related issue that distinguishes availability from accessibility of events stored in memory is dramatically supported through findings that show how dissociative memory effects can be erased by cuing. The issue of encoding and its relationship (if any) to memory consolidation, is more difficult to handle within this system but nevertheless is likely to yield ground to a joint pharmacological/ neurochemical and information-processing approach. Stated differently, the findings that emerge from comparisons of the sober vs. intoxicated state in normal subjects or alcohol abusers underline the issues that are easily dismissed when working just within some system that attempts to account for "normal" information processing. What is implied by concepts such as encoding, consolidation, the relationship between encoding and consolidation processes, notions of short-term, not so short-term memory of the distant past, and the contrasting position that emphasizes depth or elaborateness of processing episodic events might be fruitfully attacked using the intoxicated state as an experimental tool.

It also seems apparent that current notions and models posited to account for information processing in man can be more effectively studied by incorporating or attending to at least some of the biologically focused research relating brain neurochemistry and behavior. It appears clear that specific and nonspecific brain-state arousal may well play a role in modulating information storage and retrieval (McGaugh & Herz, 1972; Weingartner, Hall, Murphy, & Weinstein, 1976). Alcohol as a depressant drug does in fact alter the activity of those biogenic amines, e.g., norepinephrine, dopamine, and serotonin, in the central nervous system that modulates emotional and cognitive behaviors as well as brain-state arousal (Wallgren, 1973). Relating the neurochemical response to alcohol and its consequent effects on brain activation and arousal may well provide some important new insights about cognition in the intoxicated state. It might also serve as a useful system for studying the biology of a variety of component aspects of information flow in the interactive central nervous system.

REFERENCES

Cermak, L. S., Butters, N., & Gerrein, J. The extent of the verbal encoding ability of Korsakoff patients. *Neuropsychologia,* 1973, *11*, 85–94.

Craik, F. I. M., & Lockhart, R. S. Levels of processing: A framework for memory research. *Journal of Verbal Learning and Verbal Behavior,* 1972, *11*, 671–684.

Eich, J. E., Stillman, R. C., & Weingartner, H. Stimulus repetition and state-dependent learning. In preparation.

Eich, J. E., & Weingartner, H. Sequential retrieval strategies and dissociations of memory. In preparation.

Eich, J. E., Weingartner, H., Stillman, R. C., & Gillin, J. C. State-dependent accessibility of retrieval cues in the retention of a categorized list. *Journal of Verbal Learning and Verbal Behavior,* 1975, *14*, 408–417.

Goodwin, D. W. Two species of alcoholic "blackout." *American Journal of Psychiatry,* 1971, *127*, 1665–1670.

Goodwin, D. W., Powell, B., Bremer, D., Hoine, H., & Stern, J. Alcohol and recall: State-dependent effects in man. *Science,* 1969, *163*, 1358–1360.

McGaugh, J. L., & Herz, M. J. *Memory consolidation.* San Francisco: Albion, 1972.

Milner, B. R. Memory and the medial temporal region of the brain. In K. H. Pribram & P. E. Broadbent (Eds.), *Biology of memory.* New York: Academic Press, 1970.

Paivio, A., Yuille, J. C., & Madigan, S. A. Concreteness, imagery, and meaningfulness values for 925 nouns. *Journal of Experimental Psychology Monograph,* 1968, *76*, (1, Pt. 2).

Palermo, D. S., & Jenkins, J. J. *Word association norms. grade school through college.* Minneapolis: University of Minnesota Press, 1964.

Thorndike, E. L., & Lorge, I. *The teacher's word book of 30,000 words.* New York: Columbia University, Teachers College Press, 1944.

Tulving, E., & Thomson, D. M. Encoding specificity and retrieval processes in episodic memory. *Psychological Review,* 1973, *80*, 352–373.

Wallgren, H. Neurochemical aspects of tolerance to and dependence on ethanol. In W. M. Gross (Ed.), *Alcohol intoxication and withdrawal: Experimental Studies* I. New York: Plenum Press, 1973.

Weingartner, H. Verbal learning in patients with temporal lobe lesions. *Journal of Verbal Learning and Verbal Behavior,* 1968, *7*, 520–526.

Weingartner, H., Adefris, W., Eich, J. E., & Murphy, D. L. Encoding-imagery specificity in alcohol state-dependent learning, *Journal of Experimental Psychology: Human Learning and Memory,* 1976, *2,* 83–87.

Weingartner, H., & Faillace, L. A. Alcohol state-dependent learning in man. *Journal of Nervous and Mental Disease,* 1971, *153,* 395–406.

Weingartner, H., Hall, B., Murphy, D. L., & Weinstein, W. Imagery, affective arousal and memory consolidation. *Nature,* 1976, *263,* 311–312.

Weingartner, H., & Murphy, D. L. Brain states and memory: State-dependent storage and retrieval of information. *Psychopharmacology Bulletin,* 1977, *13*(1), 66–67.

Weingartner, H., Snyder, S. H., Faillace, L. A., & Marley, H. Altered free associations: Some cognitive effects of DOET (2, 5 dimethoxy–4–ethyl–amphetamine). *Behavioral Science,* 1970, *15,* 297–303.

Wickelgren, W. A. The long and the short of memory. *Psychological Bulletin,* 1973, *80,* 425–438.

Part V

MEMORY IN ALCOHOLICS AND KORSAKOFF PATIENTS

12

The Alcoholic Blackout
and How to Prevent It

Donald W. Goodwin

University of Kansas Medical Center

THE BLACKOUT

Definition. "Blackout," a confusing term sometimes denoting amnesia and at other times unconsciousness, has come in the alcoholism literature to designate memory loss for events that occur while drinking alcohol, where the events normally are memorable.

Prevalence and onset. Studies indicate that about two-thirds of chronic alcoholics frequently experience memory loss while drinking, but that this generally first occurs midway or late in the course of alcoholism and rarely after ingestion of moderate amounts of alcohol (Goodwin, Crane, & Guze, 1969a). Surveys of young *non*alcoholic men indicate that about one-third have experienced at least one blackout. Therefore, the notion that blackouts are an important predictor of alcoholism, as is sometimes reported in the alcoholism literature, is not supported by systematic studies. Nor, in the case of alcoholics, does it appear that blackouts often occur after ingestion of subintoxicating amounts of alcohol (in contrast to so-called pathological intoxication, which has been little studied and about which hardly anything is known [Goodwin, 1971]).

Precipitants. It is not known why some alcoholics never have blackouts, or at least have relatively mild ones, and other alcoholics experience blackouts almost every time they drink. Nor is it known why some drinkers have blackouts on some occasions and not on others, where equivalent amounts of alcohol are consumed over similar periods of time. Interview data, however, indicate that certain behaviors and historical events do have a statistical correlation with the

177

occurrence of frequent blackouts (Goodwin, Crane, & Guze, 1969b). These are:

1. Drinking large amounts *rapidly* (gulping).
2. History of frequent head injuries (heavy drinkers who were once boxers are particularly susceptible to blackouts).
3. Fatigue of physical debilitation.
4. Ingestion of hypnotics, sedatives, and tranquilizers at time of heavy drinking (Mendelson, Goodwin, Hill, & Reichman, 1976). Marijuana also may have synergistic effects with alcohol in producing memory loss.

Typology. Amnesia having a definite starting point, ending with a sense of "lost time" and involving memory loss for significant events appears to differ qualitatively from a fragmentary, spotty type of memory loss where the person only realizes that he forgot an event when told it later. Most people having frequent *en bloc* memory loss (as the former has been called) also experience the *fragmentary* kind (Goodwin et al., 1969b).

Memory loss of the en bloc type is usually total and seemingly permanent. As a rule, no amount of memory jogging, either by the person in an effort to remember or by friends telling him of the event, dispels the amnesia. Realization of having had such a blackout is often accompanied by a feeling of dread or apprehension. The person typically wonders whether he might have harmed or killed somebody.

In the case of fragmentary memory loss, at least partial return of memory is common. This may occur spontaneously or more commonly when the person is told about the forgotten event. Description of memory return is often reminiscent of "shrinkage of amnesia" said to characterize memory return after electroconvulsive therapy and concussions. The recollection has an unreal quality, "like a picture out of focus" or "like remembering a dream [Goodwin et al., 1969b, p. 1034]."

QUESTIONS ABOUT BLACKOUTS

1. Does the memory loss represent a form of registration defect? In other words, was the person in a semistuperous state or inattentive for other reasons?
2. Is the memory loss primarily psychological or physiological in origin?
3. Is the amnesia predominantly retrograde or anterograde in nature, or a mixture of both?
4. Is the blackout selective or global? In other words, are certain types of memory intact but not others?
5. Is the memory recoverable by special means such as hypnosis, amytal interview, or reingestion of alcohol?
6. Are alcoholic blackouts preventable (other than by avoidance of alcohol)?

TENTATIVE ANSWERS

1. Alcoholic blackouts have been produced under experimental conditions by giving subjects large amounts of alcohol and exposing them to normally memorable events (Goodwin, Othmer, Halikas, & Freemon, 1970). The findings indicate that the memory loss, as observed during the amnesic period, involves a specific type of memory deficit. Remote memory is apparently intact. Immediate memory (ability to remember memorable events for 1 minute) is intact. The deficit consists of a specific, short-term memory loss, defined as an inability to remember normally memorable events a short time after they occur. Predictably this is followed by inability to remember events 24 hours later. Intellectual functioning in general seems well preserved. Indeed, without formal memory testing, the short-term memory deficit may not be observable. In any case, the deficit does not appear to be based on impaired registration.

2. Is the memory loss psychologically "motivated?" In other words, does the individual forget things because he *wants* to forget them? There is no way to exclude this possibility, but studies (Goodwin et al., 1969a; Goodwin, Powell, Hill, Lieberman, & Viamontes, 1974) suggest it is not an important factor for these reasons:

a. Alcoholic subjects when asked about blackouts usually report that the forgotten events rarely were associated with guilt- or anxiety-producing behavior. Or, rather, most of the times when they had blackouts their behavior was no more or no less guilt-producing than at other times.

b. In studies where blackouts were produced under experimental conditions (5), the subjects who had blackouts behaved no differently during the blackout period than when their memory was intact. Therefore, if motivation was a factor, it was subtle and not traceable to directly observable events.

3. In many ways, the memory loss associated with acute intoxication resembles that classically identified with Korsakoff's Syndrome (Goodwin, Hill, Hopper, & Viesselman, 1975). It is mainly anterograde and occurs in people who are fully conscious, alert, and able to perform complicated tasks, despite a severe impairment of short-term memory. However, recent evidence suggests the memory loss is not global but mainly involves "semantic" memory (as opposed, say, to "acoustic" or "tactile" memory) (Cermak & Butters, 1973). A collaborative study was conducted, undertaken to determine whether blackouts similarly were selective. For methodological reasons (described elsewhere [Goodwin, 1972]), the question was not resolved; but the study did produce a serendipitous finding that will be discussed in the next section on prevention.

4. Is the memory loss reversible? As indicated earlier, the so-called en bloc memory loss appears to involve a very low degree of recoverability, if indeed any memory storage took place at all (Goodwin et al., 1969b). However, in the case

of fragmentary blackouts it was common for people to have some amount of memory recovery. Also, if asked (and sometimes when not asked), alcoholics sometimes say they lose their memory for events while drinking (such as where they hid a bottle or money), only to have the memory come back when they resume drinking again. This is reminiscent of so-called state-dependent learning in animal studies, where learning that takes place in a particular drug state is present when the animal is redrugged but not otherwise. Several studies have suggested that this also occurs, to a moderate but definite degree, in humans given alcohol (Goodwin, 1974). This has led to speculation that perhaps the alcoholic blackout is not a unitary phenomenon and that some types of memory loss may reflect state-dependent effects, the basis for which remains unknown (Goodwin, 1971).

PREVENTION

A. Provide a Prompter

As noted above, a collaborative study was conducted recently in an attempt to determine whether experimental blackouts resembled the memory loss that has recently been reported to occur in Korsakoff's syndrome (Goodwin et al., 1975). If the latter reports are borne out by further experimentation, it would appear that Korsakoff-type memory loss is selective and limited to particular "modalities." In attempts to produce experimental blackouts and simultaneously give tests that would bring out this specificity, it was discovered that the amounts of alcohol required to produce the blackouts were inconsistent with the ability to perform the tests. Therefore, we were unable to answer this question conclusively, although there was some evidence that a selective factor was indeed present.

The serendipitous finding bearing on the question of whether alcoholic blackouts are preventable came about as follows: Although the collaborative study was carefully planned, in actuality there was an apparently crucial difference in the way it was executed. The study consisted of presenting highly memorable material to intoxicated subjects at 30-minute intervals, then seeing if they could remember the material 1 minute after they were exposed to it, then again at 30 minutes, and finally 24 hours later.

In one-half of the study (conducted in St. Louis) the subjects were "cued" if they failed to spontaneously remember the usually memorable experience. Apparently as a consequence of this — this memory-prompting by use of cues — blackouts were prevented from occurring, since in 12 subjects who had histories of frequent blackouts, none had a blackout — despite blood alcohol levels in the 300 mg% range (sufficient in previous studies to produce blackouts).

On the other hand, the second group conducting the study (in Boston) produced blackouts in practically every instance.

In exploring why this difference should have occurred, it was discovered that the Boston group had *not* cued their subjects; if the subjects spontaneously failed to remember the material, the study proceeded without cuing. On the following day, they were unable to remember items that sober subjects could always remember, meeting the definition of blackout.

In other words, it would appear that blackouts *are* preventable if the drinker is constantly reminded of events that happened a short time after they happen. "Prompting" or rehearsal apparently "grooves in" the memory so that it is recoverable not only 30 minutes after the event occurs but also on the following day *if* cuing is repeated. Subjects the following day had difficulty spontaneously remembering highly memorable events, but once cued, the memory returned. In the previous study, when they had not been cued *during* the drinking period itself, cuing on the following day had no facilitative effect on recall (Goodwin et al., 1970).

B. Hormones, Drugs, and Other Chemicals

Other studies that might be performed that would have etiological implications with regard to blackouts, as well as possibly pose practical ways of preventing them, include the following:

In recent years a number of groups have found that removing the pituitary gland of rats decreased the ability of the animals to acquire conditioned avoidance behavior. Administration of ACTH, MSH, or vasopressin to the hypophysectomized rats corrected this deficiency, with the result that these animals learn nearly as well as the controls (Rigter, Van Riezen, & DeWied, 1974).

At least one group has applied this knowledge to humans in an attempt to facilitate memory in aged subjects and those who have memory impairment after electroconvulsive therapy (Miller, Kastin, Sandman, Fink, & Van Veen, 1974). Either ACTH or a fragment of ACTH — called 4-10 — was administered. The results were equivocal; whether administration of these hormones will facilitate memory remains undemonstrated. However, to our knowledge, vasopressin has not been administered, and some of the studies indicated that vasopressin was the most effective of the memory restorers. Unless contraindicated because of side effects, possibly vasopressin could be preadministered to intoxicated individuals in an attempt to prevent memory loss. It is known that alcohol inhibits vasopressin (otherwise known as antidiuretic hormone), producing diuresis. Alcohol also inhibits oxytocin, another hypothylamic hormone stored in the posterior pituitary. If these hormones are mediators of memory, possibly alcohol as an inhibitor of posterior pituitary hormones may also play a role in producing memory loss.

A third possibility would be to administer Dilantin to intoxicated individuals. The type of memory loss observed in experimental blackouts suggests that the poterior medial portions of the hippocampi may be involved, since the problem with memory "consolidation" resembles that seen in bilateral hippocampal lesioned animals, as well as in a few individuals whose hippocampi have been ablated to prevent temporal lobe seizures (Drachman & Arbit, 1966). Anticonvulsants, therefore, may have an antiseizurgenic effect that would prevent blackouts.

A further line of study deriving from recent animal data suggests that predosing animals with ascorbic acid, thiamine, and certain sulphydryl compounds may provide some protection against the toxicity of acetaldehyde, a metabolite of alcohol associated with alcohol-related ailments (Sprince, 1975). There is no direct evidence that acetaldehyde is involved in alcoholic blackouts, but thiamine deficiency is almost certainly the cause of the Wernicke—Korsakoff syndrome (Victor, 1964); and pre-dosing human subjects with large amounts of thiamine before they were given alcohol would seem to be not only a reasonable but safe procedure.

Finally, ascorbic acid in combination with reserpine apparently protects against acetaldehyde toxicity (Sprince, 1975). The depleting effect of reserpine on biogenic amines is well known, and there is a large if contradictory literature on effects of alcohol on amine levels in the brain. Again, such studies might lead to further understanding of the pathogenesis of the alcoholic blackout and also suggest ways of preventing blackouts. There has been speculation that "loss of control" and blackouts are in some way related, and preventing the blackout conceivably might aid the heavy drinker in controlling his drinking behavior (Storm & Smart, 1965).

ACKNOWLEDGMENTS

This research was supported, in part, by Alcohol, Drug Abuse, and Mental Health Administration grant DA4RG008 and Research Scientist Development Award AA-47325 (awarded to Dr. Goodwin) by the National Institute on Alcohol Abuse and Alcoholism.

REFERENCES

Cermak, L. S., & Butters, N. Information processing deficits of alcoholic Korsakoff patients. *Quarterly Journal of Studies on Alcohol*, 1973, *34*, 1110—1132.

Drachman, D. A., & Arbit, J. Is memory a multiple process? An experimental study of patients with hippocampal lesions. (Abstract) *Neurology*, 1966, *16*, 312—313.

Goodwin, D. W. Blackouts and alcohol induced memory dysfunction. *Recent Advances in Studies on Alcoholism*, Proceedings of the 1970 NIAAA Interdisciplinary Symposium, publication number (HSM) 71-9045, 1971.

Goodwin, D. W. The phenomena of alcoholic blackouts. *Proceedings, Workshop on Alcoholic Blackout,* National Institute on Alcohol Abuse and Alcoholism, 1972.

Goodwin, D. W. Alcoholic blackouts and state-dependent learning. *Federation Proceedings,* 1974, *33,* 1833–1835.

Goodwin, D. W., Crane, J. B., & Guze, S. B., Alcoholic "blackouts": A review and clinical study of 100 alcoholics. *American Journal of Psychiatry,* 1969, *126,* 191–198. (a)

Goodwin, D. W., Crane, J. B., & Guze, S. B. Phenomenological aspects of the alcoholic "blackout." *British Journal of Psychiatry,* 1969, *115,* 1033–1038. (b)

Goodwin, D. W., Hill, S. Y., Hopper, S., & Viesselman, J. O. Alcoholic blackouts and Korsakoff's Syndrome. In M. M. Gross (Ed.), *Alcohol Intoxication and Withdrawal, Experimental Studies* II. New York: Plenum Press, 1975.

Goodwin, D. W., Othmer, E., Halikas, J. A., & Freemon, F. Loss of short-term memory as a predictor of the alcoholic "blackout." *Nature,* 1970, *227,* 201–202.

Goodwin, D. W., Powell, B., Hill, S. Y., Lieberman, W., & Viamontes, J. Effect of alcohol on "dissociated" learning in alcholics. *Journal of Nervous and Mental Disease,* 1974, *158,* 198–201.

Mendelson, W. B., Goodwin, D. W., Hill, S. Y., & Reichman, J. D. The morning after: Residual EEG effects of triazolam and flurazepam, alone and in combination with alcohol. *Current Therapeutic Research,* 1976, *19,* 155–163.

Miller, L. H., Kastin, A. J., Sandman, C. A., Fink, M., & Van Veen, W. J. Polypeptide influences on attention, memory and anxiety in man. *Pharmacology Biochemistry and Behavior,* 1974, *2,* 663–668.

Rigter, H., Van Riezen, H., & DeWied, D. The effects of ACTH and vasopressin-analogues on CO_2-induced retrograde amnesia in rats. *Physiology and Behavior,* 1974, *13,* 381–388.

Sprince, H. *Federation Proceedings,* March 1, 1975, 31.

Storm, T., & Smart, R. G. Dissociation: A possible explanation of some features of chronic alcoholism and implications for treatment. *Quarterly Journal of Studies on Alcohol,* 1965, *26,* 111–115.

Victor, M. Observations on the amnestic syndrome in man and its anatomical basis. *Brain Function,* 1964, *2,* 311–340.

13
Memory Functioning in Alcoholics

Oscar A. Parsons
George P. Prigatano

*University of Oklahoma Health Sciences Center
and
Veterans Administration Hospital, Oklahoma City*

One of the common complaints by alcoholics when they finally decide to seek treatment is disturbance in memory, especially recent memory. If the alcoholism has reached the stage of diagnosable "organic brain syndrome," memory disturbance is typically present; indeed it may be one of the major symptoms leading to that diagnosis. Korsakoff's disorder with its profound memory impairment is the most notable example of such a state. But there are many other alcoholics diagnosed as having a brain syndrome that is not necessarily Korsakoff in nature. For example, in Hovarth's (1975) clinical research, 100 of 1,100 (about 9%) alcoholics presenting for treatment were diagnosed as "demented" (chronic organic brain syndrome), but only 20 of the 100 were diagnosed as having Korsakoff's disease.

Accepting a figure of about 10% of all alcoholics as having a diagnosable brain syndrome and therefore some memory impairment, what about the other 90%? There is considerable evidence that many of these alcoholics have impaired performance on tests of abstracting ability, suggestive of a mild organic syndrome (Parsons, 1975). Do these alcoholics have demonstrable memory deficits? If so, are the deficits in recent or remote memory or the retrieval processes or some combination of these? Do the deficits vary with the experimental conditions; e.g., incidental vs. intentional learning, massed vs. spaced trials, or task-relevant vs. interfering stimuli? Reviews of intellectual functioning in alcoholics do not lead to optimism about ready answers to these questions (Goodwin & Hill, 1975; Kleinknecht & Goldstein, 1972; Ryback, 1971). The fundamental questions as to the presence, kind, and extent of memory deficits in alcoholics remain to be clarified.

One of the variables most responsible for equivocal results in tests of memory function in alcoholics is that of the population sampled. In a recent paper on pneumoencephalographic findings in alcoholics, Parsons (1975) concluded that, depending upon the population studied, one could demonstrate enlarged ventricles in from 50% to 100% of the alcoholic subjects. A similar statement could be made about intellectual impairment in alcoholics. Most psychological studies of alcoholics are done in the context of treatment programs, i.e., programs where subjects are available for periods of time necessary for testing. Typically, selection procedures are undertaken that filter out individuals who may not benefit from treatment. For example, in some settings an alcoholic diagnosed as having a chronic brain syndrome would be seen as a less likely candidate for treatment than one who was not, and hence not accepted in the program. In other settings, such individuals would be retained as part of the treated group. Groups of alcoholics who vary as to number of chronic brain syndrome patients will give rise to markedly different results.

Another subject variable that we have found to be of importance is that of years of heavy drinking. In several studies we have demonstrated that short-term (less than 10 years of heavy drinking) and long-term alcoholics (10 or more years of heavy drinking) perform differently on tests of abstracting ability (Parsons, 1975). Age is another critical variable. It is well known that aging results in memory difficulties, especially when new learning is involved. There is some evidence to suggest that alcoholism may interact with age so that the older the alcoholic, the more severe the intellectual deficit, even if duration of drinking is partialed out (Jones & Parsons, 1972; Kleinknecht & Goldstein, 1972). Whether this interaction holds for memory is not known. Another variable is the high incidence of head injury in alcoholic patients (Chandler, Parsons, & Vega, 1975). Head injuries are notorious for their effect on memory. Depending on the titer of long- and short-term patients and the number of head injury patients in the sample, results on memory tests might be quite different.

Finally, one of the most important variables is the time since detoxification. Any memory investigation of alcoholics before 2 weeks have elapsed since initiating detoxification probably reflects the withdrawal condition rather than more permanent change. After the first several alcohol-free weeks, improvement in general intellectual functioning appears to be rapid in many alcoholics. Recent studies indicate that after several months of detoxification, alcoholics greatly improve their performance on cognitive tests (Goodwin & Hill, 1975; Parsons, 1977). Few studies have been carried out for longer periods of time. One of the few that retested alcoholics after 1 year found that practically no deficit remained (Long & McLachlan, 1974).

In summary, in studies of memory functioning in alcoholics, five subject variables would appear to be important to investigate: (1) the presence of a mild organic brain syndrome; (2) duration of heavy drinking; (3) age; (4) history of head injury; and (5) period of detoxification. In the subsequent sections we report on studies from our laboratory bearing on the possible effect of these variables on memory in alcoholics with the exception of the fifth variable (period of detoxification). In our studies all alcoholics have been detoxified for at least 3 weeks before testing.

As previously noted, we have demonstrated that duration of drinking and age are related to performance on abstracting tasks; in particular, the Halstead Category test and the Wisconsin Card Sorting test (WCST) (Parsons, 1975). Patients with 10 or more years of heavy drinking perform significantly more poorly than patients with less than 10 years of such drinking. Both of these tasks require that the subject solve for the principle over a series of stimulus presentations when the previous choices (both correct and incorrect) are no longer available for review. In other words, the subject must keep in memory previous choices if he is still trying to identify the principle; or if he has arrived at the correct solution, keep the principle itself in memory over trials to criterion of successful performance.

In order to look at the possible role of memory in impaired performance on such tasks, Klisz and Parsons (unpublished study) gave the Levine hypothesis testing task (Levine, 1966) to long-term ($\overline{X}$ = 14.4 years) and short-term ($\overline{X}$ = 5.0 years), old ($\overline{X}$ = 53.2 years) and young ($\overline{X}$ = 41.5 years) alcoholics. The Levine task is a concept identification type task that uses geometric forms presented visually on cards. The task for the subject is to choose one of two stimulus figures (on each trial) according to a sorting principle based on one of the attributes. The task consisted of 16 problems to be solved with 16 trials for each problem. Reinforcements were given on the 1st, 5th, 12th, and 16th trials. There were two types of presentations; the first type was similar to the other test of abstracting behavior, i.e., the stimulus presentation (card) turned over after a choice had been made; in the second type of presentation, the 16 stimulus cards were left in front of S for continued perusal with the correct choices on the reinforced trials indicated by arrows (memory-aid condition). If long-term alcoholics had greater impairment than the short-term alcoholics on the standard type of presentation and relatively less impairment on the memory-aid condition, then impaired memory could account in part for the abstracting test deficit.

The results of this experiment were surprising to us (Table 1). While the memory-aid condition resulted in significantly better performance by both groups (F = 74.31, df = 1, 36, $p < .001$), long- and short-term alcoholics did not differ in their performance. By contrast, age had a quite robust effect; older alcoholics performed significantly more poorly than younger alcoholics (F = 23.33, df = 1, 36, $p < .005$), even though the average age difference between the two groups was only about 10 years. As the short-term — long-term variable did not discriminate between groups (either as a main effect or in interactions), we then initiated another experiment with the WCST to determine whether our original findings of impaired abstracting behavior in alcoholics were repeatable.

TABLE 1
Means and Standard Deviations for Number of Correct
Solutions in Standard and Memory-Aid Conditions

Group	No. correct solutions, standard condition		No. correct solutions, memory-aid condition	
	$\bar{X}$	SD	$\bar{X}$	SD
Young short-term alcoholics (N = 10)	10.50	2.46	15.10	0.83
Young long-term alcoholics (N = 10)	10.90	2.34	13.60	1.80
Old short-term alcoholics (N = 10)	7.00	3.46	10.60	4.50
Old long-term alcoholics (N = 10)	6.10	2.38	10.10	3.36

Although this experiment is not complete, we have found that the new samples of alcoholics indeed are impaired on the WCST. However, subjects who cannot complete the WCST under standard conditions can perform it well when it is made more like a concept identification task such as Levine's test, i.e., where the relevant attributes are identified and shifts in reinforcement are announced. These findings suggest first that memory impairment in alcoholics cannot account for the differences on abstracting test performance and second, that it is in the self-initiated sets for problem solution where alcoholics have at least part of their difficulty in abstracting tasks. Finally, importance of age in tests of abstracting performance is reaffirmed. It could be argued, however, that our "memory-aid" condition within the abstracting task was not a fair or direct test. Let us therefore turn to a more specific test of possible impairment of memory, the Wechsler Memory Scale.

HEAD INJURY, ALCOHOLISM, AND MEMORY DEFICIT

A commonly used clinical psychological test of verbal memory functioning is the Wechsler Memory Scale. Wechsler (1945) designed the scale so that in a normal population memory quotients are equivalent to IQ's; e.g., a person with an IQ of 100 would have a memory quotient (M.Q.) of 100. Studies have shown lower M.Q.'s than IQ's in patients who complain of memory difficulties. These patients include Korsakoff patients (Victor, Herman, & White, 1959), head-injury patients (Black, 1973), psychomotor epileptics (Quadfasel & Pruyser, 1955), and commissurotomy patients (Zaidel & Sperry, 1974). There have been surprisingly few studies of Wechsler Memory Scale performance in alcoholics and none (to the knowledge of the authors) that controlled for or investigated the effects of head injury.

We investigated the Wechsler Memory Scale scores, Wechsler Adult Intelligence Scale IQ's, and the difference between them in four groups of patients: alcoholics with a self-reported history of head injury (H.I.); alcoholics without such a history; psychiatric patients without a history of head injury; and a group of known head-injury patients. Groups (Ns of 10 each) were matched as closely as possible on age, sex, education, handedness, race, and socioeconomic background. The groups were typically middle-aged, right-handed male patients with several years of high school education and from lower and middle social class. Patients were examined by an experienced clinician or assistants. The alcoholics were tested in the 4th and 5th week of treatment.

The results are depicted in Table 2. In column 1, the deleterious effect of head injury on memory is noted. H.I. Ss had significantly lower M.Q.'s than IQ's ($F = 5.16$, $df = 1, 36$, $p < .05$). All other groups had higher M.Q.'s than IQ's, although not significantly so. Alcoholics with head injuries had lower memory quotients than the other two non-H.I. groups, but the difference between IQ and M.Q. was not significant. A significant interaction between alcoholics vs. non-alcoholics and H.I. vs. non-H.I. was obtained ($F = 5.33$, $df = 1, 36$, $p < .05$), indicating that the effect of H.I. was greater in the nonalcoholic groups than in the alcoholic groups.

In general these findings confirm the sensitivity of the Wechsler Memory Scale to head injury. Patients who are referred to neuropsychological evaluation

TABLE 2
Wechsler IQ and M.Q. Scores

	Head injury (N = 10)	Alcoholics–head injury (N = 10)	Alcoholics–no head injury (N = 10)	Psychiatric (N = 10)
FSIQ				
X̄	92.9	95.8	98.2	106.2
SD	12.8	12.1	11.9	16.0
VIQ				
X̄	92.2	97.6	99.4	105.5
SD	12.3	12.7	11.8	17.9
PIQ				
X̄	94.1	94.0	96.8	106.9
SD	13.4	13.3	12.3	16.0
MQ				
X̄	85.9	97.4	104.2	110.0
SD	13.8	18.6	17.6	15.3
FSIQ–MQ (+100)				
X̄	107.0	98.4	94.0	96.1
SD	11.6	11.4	10.9	13.2

following brain trauma have pronounced verbal memory deficits. Although the alcoholics with head injury had the next lowest memory score, they did not show a significant IQ–M.Q. deficit. One reason for this may be in the long-standing nature of the head injury in the alcoholics. Compared to the H.I.-group average of 5.9 years duration of head injury, the alcoholics averaged 20.8 years duration. A second reason is that the H.I. patients were referred for symptoms resulting from the head injury, whereas the alcoholics were reporting head injuries that in the main had been and continued to be asymptomatic.

It is clear that the alcoholics in this study tested 4 to 5 weeks after starting treatment did not manifest a generalized decrement in memory quotient. Post hoc inspection of alcoholics' performance on various subtests of the Wechsler Memory Scale revealed, however, some interesting differences (see Table 3). Compared to the psychiatric patients ($N = 10$), the combined group of alcoholics ($N = 20$) showed significantly poorer associate-learning scores ($t = 2.72$, $p <$ .05). On both easy and hard paired-associate items, they recalled less than psychiatric patients ($t = 2.77$, $p < .01$; $t = 2.13$, $p < .05$ respectively). Also,

TABLE 3
Post Hoc Comparison of the Combined Alcoholics and Psychiatric Patients

		Alcoholics ($N = 20$)	Psychiatric ($N = 10$)	t
Wechsler Memory Scale				
Associate Learning Score	X̄	13.55	17.00	2.72[a]
	SD	3.49	2.79	
Easy score	X̄	7.88	8.70	2.77[b]
	SD	.89	.42	
Hard score	X̄	5.45	7.70	2.13[a]
	SD	2.93	2.26	
Digits total	X̄	10.80	11.50	.92
	SD	2.02	1.84	
Digits forward	X̄	6.65	6.30	.73
	SD	1.31	1.06	
Digits backward	X̄	4.15	5.20	2.21[a]
	SD	1.23	1.23	
Wechsler Adult Intelligence Scale				
Full-scale IQ	X̄	97.00	106.10	1.77
	SD	11.74	16.00	
Age	X̄	50.00	47.60	.70
	SD	6.55	12.28	
Education	X̄	10.72	12.00	1.05
	SD	2.17	3.16	

[a]$p < .05$
[b]$p < .01$
$df = 28$

although alcoholics and psychiatric patients did not differ in the numbers of digits they could recall in the forward direction (t = .73), they did differ in the recall of digits in the reverse or backward direction (t = 2.21, $p < .05$). No other significant differences were noted on other subtest scores. These findings suggest that on specific concentrational and learning tasks there may be very slight but real deficits related to that complex process called "memory." It should be stressed, however, that for all practical purposes these alcoholics had memory functioning (as measured by the Wechsler Memory Scale) appropriate to their intellectual level.

NEUROPSYCHOLOGICAL PERFORMANCE, ALCOHOLISM, AND MEMORY

We have considered duration of drinking, age, and head injury as possible factors in memory disturbances in alcoholics. Though age was found to play a definite role in memory, neither duration of drinking nor head injury (asymptomatic) had an effect. Perhaps the "memory deficit" is only present in those patients with "mild" organic brain syndromes, i.e., those patients who do not have sufficient impairment of intellectual functions as to be formally diagnosed as "organic" but who do show some impairment. To test this hypothesis we chose the Halstead–Reitan Neuropsychological Battery Impairment Index as a criterion. Numerous studies have shown the index to be sensitive to brain injury (Reitan & Davison, 1974). Alcoholics vary considerably in the degree to which they show impairment on the Halstead–Reitan battery, but in the samples to be discussed below, about 66% fall into the impaired range on the Impairment Index (Prigatano, 1977).

Will alcoholics who are impaired on the Impairment Index have memory deficits? To approach this question, 17 alcoholics with Impairment Index scores between .7 and 1.0 (moderately to severely impaired) were compared to 18 alcoholics whose Impairment Index scores were between .0 and .3 (not impaired). These subjects were asked to recall 10 words read to them over each of 10 trials in accordance with a technique described by Luria (1966). They were then distracted for a few minutes and asked to freely recall as many of the words as possible on an additional trial. The moderate to severe impairment group recalled 88.75 words over these 11 trials. The nonimpaired group recalled 95.2 words. The difference in total number of words recalled for the two groups was not significant (F = 2.68, d.f. = 1, 31, $p < .10$). Both groups had very similar learning curves as indicated by the nonsignificant groups × trials interaction ($F < 1.00$). Considering the fact that the groups were separated into extremes on the Impairment Index, the finding of a minimal and nonsignificant difference in rote, verbal memory does not support the conclusion that such memory deficits are important in abstinent alcoholics.

In these and other alcoholics, a consistent finding in our laboratory is impairment on the Halstead Speech Sounds Perception Test (Prigatano, 1977). The test consists of auditory decoding and matching of an internal memorial representation with the written choices. Perhaps short-term verbal memory is at fault in these patients. We divided 44 alcoholics into 3 groups based on their errors on the Speech Perception test. One group ($N = 15$) made 14 errors or more on the test, a performance that would be classified as moderate to severely impaired. The next group ($N = 12$) made from 8 to 13 errors, considered mildly to moderately impaired. The third group ($N = 17$) made 7 or less errors, which is considered in the nonimpaired range. The groups' mean Luria Memory scores for total recall (of 10 words over 11 trials) were respectively 85.6, 91.9, and 95.1. Although in the expected direction, these differences did not achieve significance ($F = 3.08$, $df = 2$, 41, $p < .10$). Furthermore, the learning curves were very similar for the three groups.

These findings suggest that neither overall degree of neuropsychological impairment (Impairment Index) nor specific neuropsychological impairment on a language discrimination task involving short-term memory in chronic alcoholics is related to verbal memory as measured by the Luria Word Memory Test.

MEMORY DEFICITS IN ALCOHOLICS:
A RECONSIDERATION

As noted in the beginning of this paper, memory impairment is commonly claimed by alcoholic patients presenting for treatment. Memory, especially short-term memory, has been found by a number of investigators (Jones, 1973; Ryback, 1971) to be affected by alcohol. The alcoholic, during periods of continual heavy drinking, undoubtedly has memory problems. A person who has been drinking a fifth a day for 10 years is likely to have clouding of memory sometimes called the alcoholic haze. During the period of detoxification, memory deficits are also noticeable. But after 3 or so weeks of detoxification, what evidence is there of memory impairment in nonorganic brain-syndrome patients? We are forced to conclude (happily for former alcoholics) that, if present at all, only subtle verbal memory defects exist, at least as measured by the techniques used in our studies.

Such a statement obviously does not preclude the discovery of memory deficits by use of more difficult and complex memory tasks. Some hints as to the direction of future research lie in our findings of the significantly poorer performance on Digits Backwards and on the paired-associate learning task of the Wechsler Memory Scale. Further, it is quite possible that disturbances in nonverbal memory exist in detoxified alcoholics. Prigatano (1977) has reported some interesting results on the Tactual Form Board of the Halstead Battery. Consistent with other studies, alcoholics recall the tactually perceived forms as well as control patients but are impaired on locating the forms on the form-board, i.e., recall for spatial location appears impaired. We are currently exploring this lead in our research. We are also exploring differences between long- and short-term alcoholics using some of the verbal tasks developed by Butters and Cermak (1974). In any event, the question of memory deficits in detoxified alcoholics obviously is subtle, complex, and multifaceted. At this point in our research we cannot attribute the cognitive-intellectual impairments found in alcoholics' selected neuropsychological tests to impaired memory functioning. Indeed, in detoxified alcoholics we find little to suggest that general memory functions are impaired.

ACKNOWLEDGMENTS

This research was supported in part by USPHS (NIAAA) Grant 01464. Thanks are due to Drs. David Caster and Pamela Parrish of the Alcoholism Treatment Unit of the Oklahoma City Veterans Administration Hospital for their cooperation and support. We are grateful to Mrs. Karen Dean for her help in data compilation and testing patients.

REFERENCES

Black, F. W. Cognitive memory performance in subjects with brain damage secondary to penetrating missile wounds and closed head injury. *Journal of Clinical Psychology*, 1973, *29*, 441–442.

Butters, N., & Cermak, L. S. The role of cognitive factors in the memory disorders of alcoholic patients with the Korsakoff syndrome. *Annals of the New York Academy of Sciences*, 1974, *233*, 61–75.

Chandler, B. C., Parsons, O. A., & Vega, A. Autonomic functioning in alcoholics: A study of heart rate and skin conductance. *Journal of Studies on Alcohol*, 1975, *36*, 566–577.

Goodwin, D. W., & Hill, S. Y. Chronic effects of alcohol and other psychoactive drugs on intellect, learning and memory. In J. G. Rankin (Ed.), *Alcohol, drugs and brain damage.* Toronto: Alcoholism and Drug Addiction Research Foundation of Ontario, 1975.

Hovarth, T. B. Clinical spectrum and epidemiological features of alcoholic dementia. In J. G. Rankin (Ed.), *Alcohol, drugs and brain damage.* Toronto: Alcoholism and Drug Addiction Research Foundation of Ontario, 1975.

Jones, B. M. Memory impairment on ascending and descending limbs of the blood alcohol curve. *Journal of Abnormal Psychology*, 1973, *82*, 24–32.

Jones, B., & Parsons, O. A. Specific vs. generalized deficit of abstracting ability in chronic alcoholics. *Archives of General Psychiatry*, 1972, *26*, 380–384.

Kleinknecht, R. A., & Goldstein, S. G. Neuropsychological deficits associated with alcoholism: A review and discussion. *Quarterly Journal of Studies on Alcohol*, 1972, *33*, 999–1019.

Klisz, D. K., & Parsons, O. A. Hypothesis testing in chronic alcoholics. Unpublished manuscript, 1976.

Levine, M. Hypothesis behavior by humans during discrimination learning. *Journal of Experimental Psychology*, 1966, *71*, 331–338.

Long, J. A., & McLachlan, J. F. C. Abstract reasoning and perceptual-motor efficiency in alcoholics. Impairment and reversibility. *Quarterly Journal of Studies on Alcohol*, 1974,

Luria, A. R. *Higher cortical functions in man*. New York: Basic Books, Inc., 1966.

Parsons, O. A. Brain damage in alcoholics: Altered states of unconsciousness. In M. M. Gross (Ed.), *Alcohol Intoxification and Withdrawal: Experimental Studies II*, New York: Plenum Press, 1975.

Parsons, O. A. Neuropsychological deficits in chronic alcoholics: Facts and fancies. *Alcoholism: Clinical and Experimental Research*, 1977, *1*, 51–56.

Prigatano, G. P. Neuropsychological functioning of recidivist alcoholics treated with disulfiram. *Alcoholism: Clinical and Experimental Research*, 1977, *1*, 81–86.

Quadfasel, A. F., & Pruyser, P. W. Cognitive deficit in patients with psychomotor epilepsy. *Epilepsia*, 1955, *4*, Series III, 80–90.

Reitan, R. M., & Davison, L. A. (Eds.), *Clinical neuropsychology: current status and applications*. Washington, D.C.; V. H. Winston & Sons, 1974.

Ryback, R. S. The continuum and specificity of the effects of alcohol on memory. A review. *Quarterly Journal of Studies on Alcohol*, 1971, *32*, 995–1016.

Victor, M., Herman, K., & White, E. E. A psychological study of the Wernicke–Korsakoff syndrome. *Quarterly Journal of Studies on Alcohol*, 1959, *20*, 467–479.

Wechsler, D. A standardized memory scale for clinical use. *The Journal of Psychology*, 1945, *19*, 87–95.

Zaidel, D., & Sperry, R. W. Memory impairment after commissurotomy in man. *Brain*, 1974, *97*, 263–272.

14

The Contribution of a "Processing" Deficit to Alcoholic Korsakoff Patients' Memory Disorder

Laird S. Cermak

Boston Veterans Administration Hospital
and
Boston University School of Medicine

Although alcoholic Korsakoff patients represent a very small segment within the entire population of chronic alcoholics, they have been of interest both to investigators concerned with the effects of alcohol on the central nervous system and to theorists of normal memory processes. Alcohol investigators have been interested largely because these patients have severe subcortical, deep mid-line, brain degeneration as a consequence of their long histories of alcohol consumption coupled with a thiamine deficiency; memory theorists find the patients interesting because their brain damage results in a total inability to learn and remember any new information. Evidence from investigations of these patients' memory deficit has even been cited as being perhaps the most substantial support for the classical theoretical distinction between long- and short-term memory (Cermak, 1972; Wickelgren, 1973). This is largely because of the repeated demonstration that Korsakoffs are capable of retaining a small amount of verbal information through constant rehearsal (Talland, 1965; Cermak, Reale, & DeLuca, 1977), but forget this same material rapidly as soon as rehearsal is prevented (Cermak & Butters, 1973). It is this existence of an intact processing system (STM) in the presence of a totally deficient storage system (LTM) that has been taken as evidence that STM and LTM represent two independent storage systems.

Recently, however, the distinction between STM and LTM has faded considerably in the eyes of most information processing theorists to be replaced by more contemporary multi-dimensional single trace theories that emphasize the role of initial information analysis in the determination of the probability of eventual retrieval of information (Craik & Lockhart, 1972; Cermak, 1972; Craik & Tulving, 1975). These theories might easily be extended to the problem of amnesia by proposing that amnesia is a result, at least in part, of a deficit in this initial analysis of the information. Precisely how well this assumption corresponds to the results of empirical investigation with alcoholic Korsakoff patients is the province of the present chapter. However, prior to such considerations, a more complete sketch of the "levels of processing" approach to the study of memory and a full description of these patients will be provided.

LEVELS OF PROCESSING

The dependence of verbal memory upon the analysis of incoming information has now been emphasized by a number of information-processing theorists (Atkinson & Shiffrin, 1968; Craik & Lockhart, 1972; Cermak, 1972). These theorists view memory as being a by-product of the extent of analysis an individual performs upon the information he is asked to retain. It is believed that the greater the extent of the individual's analysis, the greater the probability that he will be able to retrieve the information. The individual's analysis could potentially include the visual, phonemic and/or semantic features of the information; with the likelihood of retrieval increasing as analysis progresses from the visual to the phonemic to the semantic (Craik & Tulving, 1975). Thus, "type" of analysis is emphasized as the primary determinant of retrieval (Craik & Tulving, 1975). Any conditions (e.g., distraction, instructions, etc.) that might prevent analysis of these features, particularly at the semantic level, will act to reduce the probability that the material can be retained because the subject will be forced to rely upon an incomplete, or lower than required, analysis upon which to base his reconstruction of the information. Perhaps the most dramatic condition that might prevent such analysis would be that resulting from brain damage. Thus, an investigation of Korsakoff patients' memory and information processing can provide both a demonstration of the potential effects of chronic alcohol misuse on information processing and, also, a test of the theory that inability to retrieve is the result of impaired information analysis.

MEMORY AND PROCESSING DEFICITS

The extent of the Korsakoff patients' memory impairment has been well documented in recent years. Talland (1965) observed that these patients are unable to remember any day—to—day events, current information, or hospital personnel. Seltzer and Benson (1974) found that they could not remember any highly publicized events of recent years; although interestingly enough, they still retained a normal amount of similar information from more distant years (e.g.,

30 to 40 years ago). This older information was probably learned prior to the onset of the brain degeneration. Finally, in an analysis of a wide spectrum of these patients' memory deficits, Cermak and Butters (1973, 1975) found impairments actually existed in all three divisions of memory traditionally studied by memory investigators — namely, long-term, short-term, and sensory memory — provided that rehearsal was prevented. Thus, it is obvious that (except for recall of events from their childhood and early adulthood years) Korsakoff patients are severely deficient in every type of retentive ability available to the normal processor of information.

The possibility that these deficits might be related to impairments in feature analysis was first noted in a study reported by Cermak and Butters in 1972. In this study, a list of eight words consisting of two words from each of four categories (e.g., animals, vegetables, professions, and names), was read to the patients. Immediately following the reading of this list the patients were asked to freely recall as many of the words as they could. Then, some time later, the patients were read a similarly constructed list of eight words. However, this time they were told what the categories were going to be and were informed that they would be asked to recall each word in response to prompting by category. As can be seen in Figure 1, control subjects improved somewhat from the free to the prompted (cued) condition, but Korsakoff patients actually retrieved fewer words under cued recall than they had under free recall. While the Korsakoff patients could freely "spew-out" the words immediately after the presentation

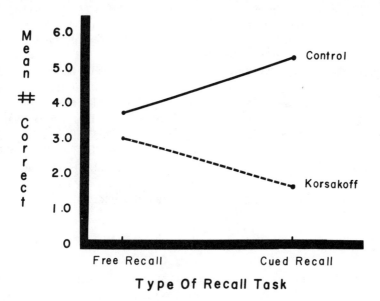

FIGURE 1   Mean number of words correctly recalled during a free recall and a cued recall task. (From Cermak & Butters, 1972, Fig. 3.)

of the list, they could not give each word back under its appropriate category. It appeared as if they were retaining the material in an uncategorized state, sufficient for immediate free recall but not for the more complex, cognitive manipulations required in cued recall. Thus, the hypothesis that impaired analysis might, in part, underlie these patients' memory difficulties began to emerge.

FALSE RECOGNITION

Further evidence supporting the hypothesis of impaired analysis in Korsakoff patients came from a study (Cermak, Butters, & Gerrein, 1973) that used an adaptation of Underwood's (1965) false recognition test. In this test, 60 words were shown to the patient at a rate of 1 word every 2 seconds; the patients' task was to detect any repetitions that occurred in the list. Though the list actually did contain repetitions, it also contained several homonyms (e.g., "bear" and "bare"), high associates ("table" and "chair"), and synonyms ("robber" and "thief"). Whenever the patient indicated that a homonym, an associate, or a synonym was a repetition, the response was scored as being a "false" recognition. The rationale of the experiment was that the more completely a patient analyzed the features of each word, the less likely he would be to falsely recognize a homonym, associate, or synonym as being a "repeat." However, if his level of analysis was meagre, he might decide that a homonym was a repeat, particularly if he was trying to rely solely upon his phonemic analysis to retain each word. It was also possible that he might indicate that an associate was a repeat, since it could have been implicitly elicited (to use Underwood's terminology) during the presentation of a prior word.

The results of this study showed that Korsakoff patients falsely recognized more homonyms and associates than the controls while, at the same time, managing to identify nearly as many actual repetitions. Like normals, however, they did not tend to make synonym or unrelated errors. This suggests that the patients must have been relying upon their phonemic analysis, coupled with a limited amount of semantic analysis (as indicated by the fact that implicit associates could not be discriminated from explicit stimuli) to retain each word. Thus, in this experiment as in the previous experiment a low level of semantic analysis was found to be characteristic of Korsakoff's syndrome.

RELEASE FROM PI

The distractor technique, another experimental paradigm, that has been used extensively in the literature on memory disorders (Milner, 1970; Baddeley & Warrington, 1973; Cermak et al., 1971, 1972), was recently adapted to study these Korsakoff patients' analytic deficits. This paradigm (Peterson & Peterson,

1959) involves presenting three words (or letters, or numbers) to the patient, followed by a task designed to prevent rehearsal of these items (counting backwards or naming colors) until recall is requested (usually 15 to 20 seconds later). Using this basic paradigm, Wickens (1970) has been able to show that proactive interference (PI) is generated by presentation of the same class of information (e.g., all animals) for several consecutive trials. This PI can be reduced by introducing material from a new class of information resulting in an increase in recall. Presumably this PI release phenomenon is a reflection of the subject's ability to analyze and store the new class of information on the basis of the features that differentiate it from the prior material. It was anticipated that the Korsakoff patients might show a release of interference when the two classes of verbal material required only a very rudimentary categorization (e.g., letters vs. numbers) but would not show a release when categorization involved more abstract semantic discriminations such as the differences in taxonomic class (e.g., animals vs. vegetables).

The first expectation was confirmed when it was found that the alpha-numeric condition did result in a PI release for the Korsakoff patients (Figure 2). In fact,

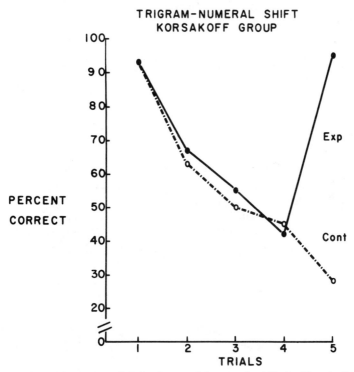

FIGURE 2 Probability of recall following an alphanumeric shift for Korsakoff patients. (From Cermak, Butters, & Moreines, 1974, Fig. 2.)

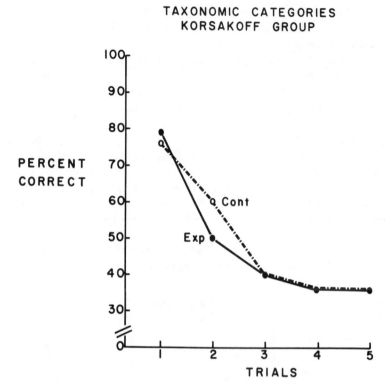

FIGURE 3 Probability of recall following a taxonomic shift for Korsakoff patients. (From Cermak et al., 1974, Fig. 3.)

their recall performance on the release trial was just as good as their performance on the first trial of the experiment. The second expectation was fulfilled when no release was found for the taxonomic shift condition (Figure 3). Here the Korsakoff patients performed at the same level following a shift in categories as they did when no switch in categories occurred. Meanwhile, a group of similarly aged, chronic alcoholics evidencing no indication of brain damage showed a release of interference following this same taxonomic shift (Figure 4). Apparently, while Korsakoff patients could detect the difference between letters and numbers and use this as the basis for keeping them separate in memory, they could not do so for the more complex, semantically-based, taxonomic categories. Thus, it was again found that Korsakoff patients were not capable of performing sufficient semantic analysis to retain verbal material, keep it free from interference in memory, and have it readily available for recall at the desired time.

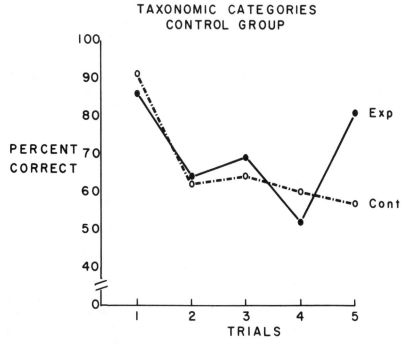

FIGURE 4 Probability of recall following a taxonomic shift for alcoholic controls. (From Cermak et al., 1974, Fig. 4).

LEVELS OF INTERFERENCE

If it is true that Korsakoff patients rely more heavily than normals upon their phonemic analysis to retain verbal information, it makes sense to assume that they would be more susceptible than normals to the effects of phonemic interference that might occur during a retention interval. Evidence that supports this assumption has been provided in a study reported by DeLuca, Cermak, and Butters (1976), using another modification of the distractor technique, in which the nature of the distractor task performed during the retention interval rather than the nature of the to-be-remembered stimulus materials was varied. In one condition of this experiment patients were asked to scan "snowflake" patterns searching for a particular configuration (a nonverbal distraction) while trying to retain three taxonomically related words; in another they were asked to shadow letters presented through headphones (acoustic distraction) while retaining the words; and in a third they were told to scan a page of words looking for words belonging to a predetermined category (which differed from that of the to-be-remembered material [semantic distraction]). As expected, the acoustic task interfered with retention of the words for the Korsakoff patients, but not for the controls; the nonverbal distraction interfered with neither group's retention, and the semantic distractor interfered with both. Thus, the Korsakoff patients must have been heavily relying upon their phonemic analysis of each word, since the acoustic task interfered so much with their retention. The semantic distractor interfered with both groups' retention; but, since it was related phonemically as well as semantically to the memoranda, it very nearly destroyed the Korsakoff patients' memory trace.

RATE OF PROCESSING

Up to this point, Korsakoff patients' analytic deficits have largely been inferred from the nature of the mistakes they made on recall and recognition tests. However, their analytic deficits have also been investigated from another vantage point, namely, by assessing the "rate" at which different types of feature analyses are performed. The rationale behind these investigations is that if Korsakoff patients are indeed impaired in their analytic abilities, then this would probably be reflected in the speed with which they could perform these analyses as well as the level they attained. A paradigm, originally developed by Posner and Mitchell (1967), was, therefore, adapted to study this possibility. Essentially the technique measures the difference between the time that it takes to decide that two letters are physically identical (e.g., A, A) and the time it takes to decide that two letters are nominally identical (e.g., A, a). This difference is believed to represent the time that it takes to analyze the phonemic features of verbal information. Using this technique, Cermak, Butters, and Moreines (1974) found that it took more time for Korsakoff patients to analyze the phonemic features of letters than it did for the chronic alcoholic controls. The Korsakoff patients' rate of information processing became notably deficient as soon as they had to perform the phonemic (nominal) analysis of the verbal material. Although the study did not show a clear-cut deficit in the analyses occurring prior to the phonemic level, a second study by Oscar—Berman, Goodglass, and Cherlow (1973) observed deficits on as basic a level as visual recognition.

In the Oscar—Berman et al. study, visual recognition thresholds for words and patterns were much higher for Korsakoff patients than they were for normal controls. In other words, the stimulus duration had to be longer before the Korsakoff patients could identify the word than was the case for the controls. In addition, these investigators found that the "masking" effect of a second stimulus upon the identification of the first was present at longer intertrial intervals for the Korsakoff patients than it was for controls. These findings were interpreted as indicating that Korsakoff patients' rate of analyzing the visual features of a stimulus is slower than normals. Thus, the patients analyze both the physical and phonemic features of verbal information at a rate slower than that performed by normals — which, understandably, places them at a distinct disadvantage in the amount of analysis they can accomplish within any given time.

RATE OF RETRIEVAL

Once it became evident that the rate at which Korsakoff patients "analyze" incoming verbal information is impaired, it seemed reasonable to investigate whether or not other aspects of their information-processing system were similarly affected. The most logical candidate for assessment became the rate at which Korsakoff patients could retrieve information known to exist in storage. The paradigm that was selected as appropriate for this investigation was one developed by Sternberg (1966) in which a short list of letters (two to six) is presented to the patient, followed immediately by a probe letter. The patient must decide whether or not this letter was a member of the just-presented set and indicate this decision by depressing either a predesignated "yes" key or "no" key. The keys are programmed to terminate a timer that was activated by the presentation of the probe. That Korsakoff patients "knew" the set of letters prior to the probe was evidenced by the fact that they responded correctly almost 100% of the time. However, their rate of responding was slower than normals in two respects (see Figure 5). First, the slope of the line plotting reaction time as a function of the serial position of the target stimulus was steeper for the Korsakoffs than it was for the normals. This indicated that they were scanning the list they had memorized more slowly than were the controls. Second, the intercept of the same line at the Y-axis was higher for the Korsakoff patients than for normals. This meant that each individual stimulus in the list was being checked against the probe item more slowly for Korsakoffs than for normals. Both these measures thus suggested that Korsakoff patients are retarded in their speed of retrieval when compared with normal rates.

Another speed-of-retrieval task performed with these patients produced essentially the same conclusion. Butters, Cermak, Jones and Glosser (1975) found that Korsakoff patients were capable of detecting instances when particular numbers were presented to them through headphones, but were deficient when a particular combination of numbers had to be detected (e.g., in the instance of a dichotic simultaneous presentation of a 5 in one ear and a 9 in the other). However, when the interpair interval was increased from 1.2 seconds to 2 seconds, the Korsakoff patients performed normally. Apparently, Korsakoff patients simply needed more time than normals to read out the material held in sensory store. When the pairs of stimuli occurred too rapidly, each essentially masked this readout from sensory store and the patients' performance was impaired.

These two experiments suggest that Korsakoff patients' rate of immediate retrieval of verbal information is significantly slower than it is for normals. This,

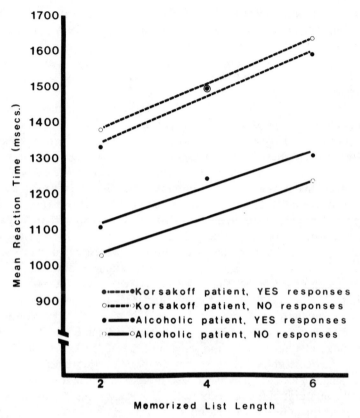

FIGURE 5 The relation between recognition–response latency and set size for alcoholic Korsakoff and alcoholic control patients (From Naus, Cermak, & DeLuca, in press, Fig. 1.)

coupled with their impaired rate of initial analysis, helps to explain why they have so much trouble learning and remembering new information. Thus far, though, little has been mentioned about their nonverbal retention. This is because it is much more difficult to perform as complete an analysis of nonverbal retention, since little to nothing is known about nonverbal "levels" of processing even in normal memory. Nevertheless, one study in particular has given us a feel for the problems these patients must experience in the nonverbal realm.

NONVERBAL RETENTION

One of the few major investigations of nonverbal retention of Korsakoff patients has recently been performed by Cermak, Reale, and DeLuca (1977), who utilized the Peterson distractor technique with nonverbal materials. Patients were shown a randomly generated visual form and then, following a retention interval, where shown the same or a different form and asked to respond "same" or "different." In some cases the distractor task consisted of searching other visual patterns for a match of a target item; in others the interval was unfilled. It was discovered that nonverbal retention dissipated rapidly when the distractor occurred and gradually when the interval was unfilled. In contrast, verbal material dissipated gradually when verbal distraction occurred during the retention interval and not at all when no distraction occurred (see Figure 6).

Evidently, Korsakoff patients can rehearse verbal materials using a form of acoustic rehearsal based upon their phonemic analysis of the information, but they cannot do anything similar with nonverbal information. In addition, whatever mechanism these patients use to rehearse verbal material must also strengthen the trace sufficiently to permit retrieval for seconds after the re-

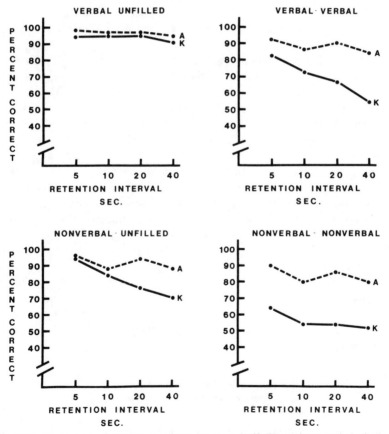

FIGURE 6 Percentage of correct responses by Korsakoff (K) patients and alcoholic (A) controls on two verbal and two nonverbal STM distractor paradigm recognition tasks. (From Cermak, Reale, & DeLuca, 1977, Fig. 1.)

hearsal ceases. On the other hand, lack of such a recirculatory mechanism for nonverbal materials results in no such strengthening, and immediate retention loss consequently occurs.

EVALUATION OF
THE "LEVELS OF PROCESSING" APPROACH

The bulk of the evidence that has been presented here indicates that alcoholic Korsakoff patients exhibit deficits in their initial processing of verbal information. It has been shown that these patients process even the most rudimentary levels more slowly and less completely than normals and — even when given sufficient time for analysis — seem to prefer relying upon phonemic recirculation rather than semantic analysis. Their slower processing speed may dictate this preference; but, regardless of cause, such reliance upon phonemic analysis results in a less permanent memory trace than that which occurs when semantic analysis is utilized. As a consequence these patients are at a distinct disadvantage when retrieval is required.

This semantic deficit should not be taken to mean that Korsakoff patients are impaired in their linguistic abilities. Indeed they seem to have as good a grasp of vocabulary and utilization of speech as any individuals with their age and background (Cermak, 1977). Instead it seems to be the case that they simply do not or cannot use this storehouse of information to analyze new incoming information as well as normal. Feature analysis of incoming information may well be impaired, because the comparison of new features with those already in memory cannot be performed rapidly or adequately.

The levels of analysis theory appears to have stood the test with amnesic patients quite well, at least for verbal retention. When more is understood about normal levels of nonverbal analysis perhaps parallel findings will be found to exist for Korsakoffs in this area as well. The results that have been reported here do not, of course, completely obviate the STM–LTM dichotomy introduced at the onset of this chapter; but they do suggest that the alternative to this dichotomy — namely, levels of processing — is capable of encompassing the results from studies on amnesia. The use of this framework with amnesics has proven valuable in contributing to our understanding of the factors underlying memory deficits; and, in return, the findings with amnesics has led to a further understanding of normal human memory.

EXTENDING THIS APPROACH TO
CHRONIC ALCOHOLICS' MEMORY DIFFICULTIES

What seems to be needed at this time is an extension of the "levels of processing" approach outlined in this paper to the study of memory difficulties seen in non-Korsakoff, chronic alcoholics. It may well be that subtle analytic deficits exist, and can be assessed, in chronic alcoholics using information-processing paradigms. This may be most evident, as suggested by Cermak and Ryback (1976), in older alcoholics following drinking episodes because of the effects of alcohol on the aging brain. But subtle deficits may begin to appear in much younger alcoholics and could be used as diagnostic indices. It may also be the case that the "blackout" state described by Goodwin (1972) results from a temporary cessation of information processing, rendering the intoxicated alcoholic not unlike a Korsakoff. Evidence to favor this notion was informally documented during the informal co-investigation this author performed with Goodwin (this volume). Alcoholics under the blackout conditions performed analytic tasks on a level comparable to Korsakoffs. Finally, state dependency might well be the result of analysis performed under one state resulting in a type of storage that can only be tapped in the presence of the same stimulus conditions. These, of course, represent only a few of the wide variety of alcoholic conditions that might be investigated using the "levels of processing" approach. In light of the success obtained using this approach with Korsakoff patients, it would appear that such a framework would be equally productive in these other areas.

ACKNOWLEDGMENTS

The research included in this report was supported in part by a NIAAA Grant AA–00187 to Boston University School of Medicine and by the Medical Research Service of the Veterans Administration.

REFERENCES

Atkinson, R. C., & Shiffrin, R. M. Human memory: A proposed system and its control processes. In K. W. Spence and J. T. Spence (Eds.), *The psychology of learning and motivation.* Vol. 2. New York: Academic Press, 1968.

Baddeley, A. D., & Warrington, E. K. Memory coding and amnesia. *Neuropsychologia,* 1973, *11,* 159–165.

Butters, N., Cermak, L. S., Jones, B., & Glosser, G. Some analyses of the information processing and sensory capacities of alcoholic Korsakoff patients. In M. M. Gross (Ed.), *Alcohol Intoxication and Withdrawal:* Experimental Studies II, New York: Plenum Press, 1975.

Cermak, L. S. *Human memory: Research and theory.* New York: Ronald Press, 1972.

Cermak, L. S. The development and demise of verbal memory. In A. Caramazza & E. Zurif, (Eds.), *The acquisition and breakdown of language: Parallels and divergencies.* Baltimore: The Johns Hopkins Press, 1977.

Cermak, L. S., & Butters, N. The role of interference and encoding in the short-term memory deficits of Korsakoff patients. *Neuropsychologia,* 1972, *10,* 89–95.

Cermak, L. S., & Butters, N. Information processing deficits of alcoholic Korsakoff patients. *Quarterly Journal of Studies on Alcohol,* 1973, *34,* 1110–1132.

Cermak, L. S., & Butters, N. The role of language in the memory disorders of brain damaged patients. The New York Academy of Sciences Conference on Origins and Evolution of Language and Speech, New York, September 1975.

Cermak, L. S., Butters, N., & Gerrein, J. The extent of the verbal encoding ability of Korsakoff patients. *Neuropsychologia*, 1973, *11*, 85–94.

Cermak, L. S., Butters, N., & Goodglass, H. The extent of memory loss in Korsakoff patients. *Neuropsychologia*, 1971, *9*, 307–315.

Cermak, L. S., Butters, N., & Moreines, J. Some analyses of the verbal encoding deficit of alcoholic Korsakoff patients. *Brain and Language*, 1974, *1*, 141–150.

Cermak, L. S., Reale, L., & DeLuca, D. Korsakoff patients' nonverbal vs. verbal memory: Effects of interference and mediation on rate of information loss. *Neuropsychologia*, 1977, *15*, 303–310.

Cermak, L. S., & Ryback, R. Recovery of verbal short-term memory in alcoholics. *Journal of Studies on Alcohol*, 1976, *37*, 46–52.

Craik, F. I. M., & Lockhart, R. S. Levels of processing: A framework for memory research. *Journal of Verbal Learning and Verbal Behavior*, 1972, *11*, 671–684.

Craik, F. I. M., & Tulving, E. Depth of processing and the retention of words in episodic memory. *Journal of Experimental Psychology: General*, 1975, *104*, 268–294.

DeLuca, D., Cermak, L. S., & Butters, N. The differential effects of semantic, acoustic and nonverbal distraction on Korsakoff patients' verbal retention performance. *International Journal of Neurosciences*, 1976, *6*, 279–284.

Goodwin, D. W. The phenomena of alcoholic blackouts. *Proceedings, Workshop on Alcoholic Blackouts,* National Institute on Alcohol Abuse and Alcoholism, 1972.

Milner, B. Memory and the medial temporal region of the brain. In K. H. Pribram & D. E. Broadbent (Eds.), *Biology of memory*. New York: Academic Press, 1970.

Naus, M. J., Cermak, L. S., & DeLuca, D. Retrieval processes in alcoholic Korsakoff patients. *Neuropsychologia*, in press.

Oscar–Berman, M., Goodglass, H., & Cherlow, D. G. Perceptual laterality and iconic recognition of visual materials by Korsakoff patients and normal adults. *Journal of Comparative and Physiological Psychology*, 1973, *82*, 316–321.

Peterson, L. R., & Peterson, M. J. Short-term retention of individual verbal items. *Journal of Experimental Psychology*, 1959, *58*, 193–198.

Posner, M. I., & Mitchell, R. F. Chronometric analysis of classification. *Psychological Review*, 1967, *74*, 392–409.

Seltzer, B., & Benson, D. F. The temporal pattern of retrograde amnesia in Korsakoff's disease. *Neurology*, 1974, *24*, 527–530.

Sternberg, S. High speed scanning in human memory. *Science*, 1966, *153*, 652–654.

Talland, G. A. *Deranged memory*. New York: Academic Press, 1965.

Underwood, B. J. False recognition produced by implicit verbal responses. *Journal of Experimental Psychology*, 1965, *70*, 122–129.

Wickelgren, W. A. The long and the short of memory. *Psychological Bulletin*, 1973, *80*, 425–438.

Wickens, D. D. Encoding categories of words: An empirical approach to meaning. *Psychological Review*, 1970, *77*, 1–15.

Author Index

Numbers in *italics* refer to pages on which the complete references are listed.

Subject Index

217